Debating Human Genetics

Debating Human Genetics is based on ethnographic research focusing primarily on the UK publics who are debating and engaging with human genetics, and related bio and techno-science. Drawing on recent interviews and data, collated in a range of public settings, it provides a unique overview of multiple publics as they 'frame' the stake of the debates in this emerging, complex and controversial arena.

The book outlines key sites and applications of human genetics that have sparked public interest, such as biobanks, stem cells, genetic screening and genomics. It also addresses the 'scientific contoversies' that have made considerable impact in the public sphere – the UK police DNA database, gene patenting, 'saviour siblings' and human cloning. By grounding the concepts and issues of human genetics in the real life narratives and actions of patient groups, genetic watchdogs, scientists, policy makers and many other public groups, the book exemplifies how human genetics is a site where public knowledge and value claims converge and collide, and identifies the emergence of 'hybrid publics' who are engaging with this hybrid science.

Alexandra Plows is a Research Fellow with The Wales Institute of Social and Economic Research, Data and Methods (WISERD), Bangor University. Her research has focused on different types of public engagement in controversial arenas including the environment, globalisation and technoscience; an overview is provided in a recent paper in *Sociology Compass*.

Genetics and Society

Series Editors: Paul Atkinson, *Distinguished Research Professor in Sociology, Cardiff University*, Ruth Chadwick, *Director of Cesagen, Cardiff University*, Peter Glasner, *Professorial Research Fellow for Cesagen, Cardiff University*, Brian Wynn, *Associate Director of Cesagen, Lancaster University*

The books in this series, all based on original research, explore the social, economic and ethical consequences of the new genetic sciences. The series is based in the ESRC's Centre for Economic and Social Aspects of Genomics, (Cesagen) the largest UK investment in social-science research on the implications of these innovations. With a mix of research monographs, edited collections, textbooks and a major new handbook, the series will be a major contribution to the social analysis of new agricultural and biomedical technologies.

Series titles include:

Governing the Transatlantic Conflict over Agricultural Biotechnology
Contending coalitions, trade liberalisation and standard setting
Joseph Murphy and Les Levidow

New Genetics, New Social Formations
Peter Glasner, Paul Atkinson and Helen Greenslade

New Genetics, New Identities
Paul Atkinson, Peter Glasner and Helen Greenslade

The GM Debate
Risk, politics and public engagement
Tom Horlick-Jones, John Walls, Gene Rowe, Nick Pidgeon, Wouter Poortinga, Graham Murdock and Tim O'Riordan

Growth Cultures
Life sciences and economic development
Philip Cooke

Human Cloning in the Media
Joan Haran, Jenny Kitzinger, Maureen McNeil and Kate O'Riordan

Local Cells, Global Science
Embryonic stem cell research in India
Aditya Bharadwaj and Peter Glasner

Handbook of Genetics and Society
Paul Atkinson, Peter Glasner and Margaret Lock

Debating Human Genetics

Contemporary issues in public policy
and ethics

Alexandra Plows

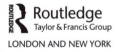
Routledge
Taylor & Francis Group

LONDON AND NEW YORK

First published 2011
by Routledge
2 Park Square, Milton Park, Abingdon, Oxon, OX14 4RN

Simultaneously published in the USA and Canada
by Routledge
270 Madison Avenue, New York, NY 10016

Routledge is an imprint of the Taylor & Francis Group, an informa business

Typeset in Times New Roman by Newgen Imaging Systems (p) Ltd,
Chennai, India
Printed and bound in Great Britain by TJ International Ltd, Padstow,
Cornwall

British Library Cataloguing in Publication Data
A catalogue record for this book is available from the British Library

Library of Congress Cataloging in Publication Data
Plows, Alexandra.
Debating human genetics : contemporary issues in public policy and ethics/
by Alexandra Plows.
p. cm.
1. Medical genetics–Moral and ethical aspects–Great Britain. 2. Human
genetics–Moral and ethical aspects–Great Britain. 3. Medical genetics–
Research–Methodology–Great Britain. 4. Human genetics–Research–
Methodology–Great Britain. 5. Medical genetics–Government policy–
Great Britain. 6. Human genetics–Government policy–Great
Britain. I. Title.
RB155.P566 2010 2011
362.196'04200941–dc22
2009052326

ISBN 13: 978-0-415-45109-3 (hbk)
ISBN 10: 0-415-45109-4 (hbk)

ISBN 13: 978-0-415-45110-9 (pbk)
ISBN 10: 0-415-45110-8 (pbk)

ISBN 13: 978-0-203-92692-5 (ebk)
ISBN 10: 0-203-92692-7 (ebk)

Contents

Acknowledgements

To Gareth and Seren, from the bottom of my heart, for their love, support and patience. Huge thanks to Sarah Sexton for sticking with me and the process from first to final draft, and for all her advice and support, and to Susan Hogben for the major surgery to chapter 5. My thanks also to Helen Wallace, Joan Haran, Kean Birch, Michael Reinsborough and Ian Rees-Jones for their input and work on various chapter drafts at short notice. Many thanks to Peter Glasner for extremely helpful and constructive comments on the draft MS, and to Graham Day for proofreading some of the draft. I am extremely grateful to David Alden for the very time consuming and pains-taking work which he undertook chasing up endnotes and bibliographical references. Diolch i Rhys Trimble, for writing the scientific glossary. Thanks to the editorial team at Routledge, in particular Gerhard Boomgaarden, for their patience with what turned out to be a long process, and thanks also to Helen Greenslade. Thanks to the 'Women in Biotechnology' conference, Rome 2007, organisers and participants, in particular to Giovanna di Chiro, Susanne Uusitalo, Wendy Harcourt and Marsha Darling, whose friendship and insights have inspired me greatly. Thanks to my PIs on the 'Emerging Politics' project, Ian Welsh and Rob Evans. Especial thanks to all my inter-viewees and all the people whose expertise informed the research on which this book is based. I sincerely hope to have done justice to the perspectives and knowledge bases I encountered. Thanks also to my friends and collea-gues, too many to mention individually, for your advice, input and support. To all the above I am indebted; the book would not have been written with-out you. Any errors in the text are mine.

Introduction

This is a book about how and why different sorts of publics, predominantly in the UK, are debating, engaging with, human genetics[1] and what they are saying and doing. Human genetics is impacting on the public sphere in many different settings, in specific contexts such as genetic testing, and is increasingly the catalyst for public engagement. People tend to construct – 'frame' – human genetics in terms of their existing personal points of view, their political and cultural frameworks, their 'lifeworlds' (Habermas 1987). They encounter human genetics as individuals, as members of different campaign groups and communities, through policy initiatives, through the media and so on. Drawing on project work during 2003–7, the book provides situated examples of how different publics in Britain are encountering and framing the debates on 'human genetics'.

The theory of framing was first developed by Goffman (1974). A 'frame' is

> an interpretive schemata that simplifies and condenses the 'world out there' by selectively punctuating and encoding objects, situations, events, experiences, and sequences of action within one's present and past environment.
>
> (Snow and Benford 1992: 137)

In other words, people, groups, networks and institutions develop 'frames' – ways of constructing the world – based on pre-existing values, and ways of doing things, and adapt these frames in a process of constructing meanings for things in the present moment; when faced with a specific issue, people will 'frame' it in their own way. For example, here is 'Alice' 'framing' human genetics:

> if people feel they have to get to know all the science ... then what's going to happen is people get bogged down in [it] ... But ... the issue isn't the science it's the inequality ... the humanitarian ... issues.
>
> ('Alice')

Frames are works in progress, constantly co-constructed. This book identifies and analyses how, why, where and when different social actors are debating – 'framing' – human genetics; what stakes people raise when they engage with specific issues and applications; what it is that matters to them. This includes an analysis of how debates are set up in specific circumstances and how different publics are involved in or respond to this process; how they are seeking to challenge, and to re-frame, debates which have been set up, for example, through policy frameworks.

In identifying and understanding public engagement with human genetics, the book differentiates between two typologies of public engagement. Informed by theories of deliberative democracy (Habermas 1987; Dryzek 2000; Fischer 2000) and by social movement theory (Diani 1992; Melucci 1996), the book differentiates between public engagement as a certain type of '*policy practice*', and public engagement as '*social movement*', whereby publics take action and frame issues on their own terms, generally outside the policy sphere. Thus, a running theme throughout the book is the question of what public engagement *is*, and what it is *for*.

Public engagement as a policy process is about the 'democratic governance' of technologies, part of what Dryzek (2000) terms a 'strong' deliberative democracy, and described in terms of hierarchical 'tree-like' structures by Deleuze and Guattari (1987). Such top-down policy formats mean that publics encounter issues already framed through the lens of governance, as they are rolled out as part of regulatory structures. A key issue is what is put in or left out of this process and how this affects the sorts of debates which are had, the sorts of issues which are discussed, and the sorts of publics – stakeholders – which engage in them. The book provides different case study examples of public engagement as policy practice, and public responses. For example, the policy-orientated move towards 'upstream public engagement' (Wilsden and Willis 2004; Wynne 2006), which aims to proactively engage with stakeholders 'upstream' as a move towards what might be termed 'best practice' in public engagement, has been criticised as still being, relatively speaking, an 'end of pipe' process in terms of the still-limited ability of 'the public' to impact on the agenda-setting process. For example, the following definition of public consultation was given in a Cabinet Office document:

> Consultation is … a form of engagement that is appropriate when the policy process is already underway and there is an intention to make changes or deliver specific outcomes. It therefore does not invite an open debate on very broad areas of public policy, nor does it empower those who participate with the final decision.
>
> (Cabinet Office 2007: 7)

In some cases as a deliberate response to perceived inadequacies in the framing of policy-led public engagement debates, many different sorts of publics are engaging outside the policy process, for example through networking, capacity-building events such as workshops, and protest events. Such forms of public engagement, defined in this book as 'social movement', involve different publics framing the stakes of debate on their own terms. This is public engagement as grassroots, self-initiated forms of mobilisation, catalysed not just by the specific issues at stake but also, often, a critique of governance; power relations and agenda setting. Such publics are shown to be consciously 'tilting the frame' (Steinberg 1998), 'challenging codes' (Melucci 1996), enabling issues to be seen in a different perspective, having a different debate. Here 'Lucy' expresses her frustration with the policy process as it stands: 'the [stem cell] debate has been framed in a certain way, you're either for or against ... so other issues, other considerations ... cannot be expressed' ('Lucy').

Social movements – and other sorts of social networks – operate through fluid network activity, disseminating information, constructing identities, and developing sets of meanings, or frames (Diani 1992). These interactive, organic, horizontal (that is, non-hierarchical) network processes have been defined as 'rhizomic' (Deleuze and Guattari 1987). Public engagement can thus also be understood in terms of network relationships between individuals and groups. Catalysed by specific circumstances, boundaries blur between different public groups, social spheres and roles, to form 'hybrid' clusters of different sorts of publics, for example the mix of policy makers, scientists and 'stakeholders' who make up a specific advisory board. Importantly, therefore, such hybridisation can encompass both the informal, 'rhizomic' grassroots activity of social networks, and more formalised, institutional, policy-orientated activity. These social network convergences have been termed 'assemblages' (Irwin and Michael 2003). In the right circumstances, such convergences can enable resources such as knowledge claims to be transferred across networks enabling 'cross talk' (Bucchi 2004) to occur across social boundaries, for example between 'scientists' and 'activists'.

A particular type of method, known as ethnography or participant observation (chapter 1) facilitated the identification of a broader range of UK publics who were engaging with human genetics outside the radar of the policy process, showing how these publics are framing the issues in their own terms: framed in banners, in the titles of workshops, in the ways in which issues are framed in discussions by workshop participants. Ethnography is thus argued to be an important form of 'upstream public engagement', in that it can identify emergent, plural, ambivalent accounts in 'messy' social fields – complex and ambivalent arenas. It can provide accounts of what 'Lucy' terms 'the other considerations' being expressed by different publics, and show how this complements public engagement as policy practice, by highlighting a broader range of debates being had about human genetics.

Who are 'the public'?

Human genetics is emergent territory where even those who are most aware of what is happening are still grappling with defining the stakes. The book focuses on some of the 'interest groups' (Tait 2001) who are alert, for a number of reasons, to emergent issues and so among the first to engage with them. These can be defined as 'prime movers' (McAdam 1986) and 'early risers' (Tarrow 1998), who engage with the stakes of the debate early on and who are key to how issues are 'framed'. In this regard policy makers are clearly also public 'prime movers'. The book also identifies that many members of 'the general public' are also engaging with human genetics in different ways, and that this is set to increase dramatically in the future. This is because 'the public' is not only willing and able to engage with publicly held debates, for example, over the creation of 'saviour siblings'; they are also increasingly likely to encounter human genetics personally in the form of a specific technological application – for example, being offered a genetic test for carrier status for a specific disease or condition, or being asked to donate DNA to the UK Biobank, or encountering the sale of online genetic test kits. The blurring of categories such as consumer and patient is a rapidly emergent, and important, trend, discussed further in chapters 4 and 5.

While the book does aim to address the question of what public engagement is and by implication who 'the public' are, in no way is it intended to be definitive about what sorts of publics there are, or indeed about what the stakes of the debates are or could be. Inevitably, while showing how the debates are 'framed' by certain publics in certain ways and how other publics are trying to re-frame the debates, the book itself contributes to 'framing' the debate, by focusing on certain groups and certain issues. This is an inevitable problem to which the only solution is methodological reflexivity. This book aims simply to be a further contribution to the ways in which publics in a range of different settings, as well as social science and other disciplines, are interrogating what sorts of other debates about human genetics are being, or might potentially be, had. And also, where one might look for them.

'Public engagement with human genetics' is complex, and as such is characterised by complex network activity which often results in the creation of hybrid 'assemblages'. Some of these are quite formal and institutionalised, such as a range of civil society perspectives enrolled onto the advisory committee of the Human Genetics Commission. Other sorts of 'assemblages' are extremely informal, fluid and shifting, consisting of network relationships and occasionally focused campaign activity. Temporary campaign alliances, for example, formed between certain UK feminists in 2006/7 in relation to concern about the sourcing and use of women's eggs for stem cell research. Case study examples of these social assemblages are provided in different chapters. In identifying some of these assemblages, and through an analysis of the sorts of issues raised by these different publics, the book gives an account of the social framing of complexity and ambivalence – human genetics 'beyond pro and anti'.

Significantly, as well as forming assemblages, publics do also clash with each other, drawing lines, and these 'line drawing' debates are generally what get heard most loudly in the public sphere, as the book demonstrates in different contexts. Often it is the 'usual suspects', individuals and groups, who are actors in a publicly staged morality play, whereby all issues are framed into a 'pro or anti' debate. These can happen because of moral absolute positions, perhaps the most pervasive being pro-life and religious moral positioning of 'the rights of the embryo' above all else. A strong voice amongst many of the multiple publics mobilising over human genetics comes from patient groups who wish for cures and treatments for disease. Further, specific cultural and political frameworks lean towards this type of 'for or against' model; it is difficult to mobilise media space to articulate complexity, and much easier to tell 'black and white' stories, and to enrol larger than life actors – 'expert scientists', for example. UK political debating culture, informed by the UK legal system, works essentially on a 'for or against' model. Accordingly, many public debates and policy-initiated public consultations on human genetics, biotechnology and associated reproductive technologies, are framed within this pro or anti format.

The book highlights a broad range of public positions and issues which are often drowned by these loudly heard, often polarised, debates; identifying instead how many people in fact display ambivalence and a reflexive awareness that issues are often more complex than being 'for or against' stem cell research, for example. Throughout the book, examples are given of how some human genetics debates have been framed in polarising 'for or against' ways, emphasising how it is this framing which is itself the subject of contestation, as 'Andy' highlights: 'the debate is framed as a simple binary opposition ... it's painful to try and explain the nuances ... '('Andy', genetics watchdog spokesperson, during Cesagen conference, UK, 2004).

'Andy', like other prime movers, consistently identifies specific socialised manifestations of political power, where policy makers and scientific 'experts' co-construct a space within which dissent is difficult to articulate and often de-legitimised, or where issues are simply not enrolled as relevant stakes for discussion. This again returns to the issue of what public engagement *is* and what it is *for*.

It is of course very important to identify when people draw 'lines in the sand'; this boundary drawing is happening in multiple contexts, sometimes in predictably polarised clashes, and sometimes in more negotiated stakes-setting in emergent debates. These boundary-drawing activities and discourses can also be understood as types of network relationships between different groups and individuals. Line drawing, ring fencing and boundary marking are important repertoires used by all who engage with debates on human genetics, and are especially important when issues are new and actors are grappling with emergent, and complex, stakes. For example, when in 2006/7 the HFEA (Human Fertilisation and Embryology Authority) supported the donation of human eggs for stem cell lines, this was a 'line in the sand' moment for many feminist academics and others, who publicly criticised the circumstances under which eggs could be taken from women's bodies (Plows 2008b, chapter 2). This did *not*, however, mean that these feminists were 'anti stem cell research' per se.

Overview of content: chapter summaries

The story of the different publics engaging with 'human genetics' is inextricably connected with the story of specific human genetics technologies and applications as they emerged onto the public stage in a specific timeframe. The book provides some snapshots of some key moments, giving an overview of the sorts of issues which were generating public debate, such as the developments in human embryonic stem cell research and the UK Biobank. Here the book draws on the author's own self-assembled sets of knowledge claims about 'the science itself', drawn primarily from key informants interviewed during the course of the project, and from a range of other sources including the media, specific science websites, policy publications, patient group and watchdog websites, and so on; in other words, the data sources themselves. The book's explanation of 'the science', then, is itself very much a socially constructed product;[2] the book has aimed to identify some of the knowledge claims about 'the science itself' and some of the knowledge claims about 'what the science *means*'. This is a difficult feat to pull off, not least because 'the science' changes so fast, and the meanings of scientific terms themselves are contested and complex territory. All chapters provide an overview of 'the science' and its potential or actual applications; and accompanying public commentary from a variety of sources, in particular from 'prime movers'. Each chapter also gives situated examples of how 'assemblages' of fluid, hybrid publics are forming to respond to 'human genetics' as they identify and frame emerging issues. There are shown to be many convergences between the issues identified in different chapters and these convergences are also catalysing the network relationships between multiple publics.

Chapter 1 further interrogates what is meant by 'public engagement', reiterating the difference between public engagement as social movement, and public engagement as policy practice. Social Movement Theory tools and principles are introduced, showing how these tools have have informed both the definition of public engagement with human genetics, and the accompanying methodology for mapping it. Hybrid, plural and grassroots publics are shown to be engaging in many different contexts. This first section also provides examples of the sorts of public engagement mapped during the research. Second, the chapter discusses the qualitative methods used to provide and analyse the data in this book, such as ethnography and interviews. The chapter then introduces the two case study sites which were the core focus of qualitative research; environmental social justice and Disability Rights groups (defined here as 'sustainability citizenship' networks), who for various reasons tend to be cautious about or critical of human genetics applications; and patient groups and their supporters, who tend to be extremely supportive of them. Other civil society groups who are engaging in the debates are introduced, noting that scientists, policy makers and the media are also key 'prime movers'. An overview of 'the general public' and how 'the general public' engages, or could engage, with human genetics provides further reflections on concepts of hybrid civil society.

Chapters 2–5 give more detailed accounts of how these different publics have engaged with some specific human genetics issues and applications which were catalysing a great deal of social activity during the research timeframe. Chapter 2 provides a narrative account of stem cell research in general, human embryonic stem cell (hESC) research in particular, and a case study focus on UK HFEA legislation in 2006 regarding the sourcing of human eggs. It identifies what research has been carried out and what the expectations of the science are; namely cures and treatments for named diseases such as Huntington's disease. The chapter gives examples of key public debates, identifying the sorts of issues which have catalysed debate, how these issues have been 'framed', and by whom. Narratives of public engagement are provided; discourses of hope and opposition relating to the use of the human embryo are common frames amongst patient groups and pro-lifers. However, others such as UK feminists are framing a more complex and ambivalent set of risks and concerns relating to the use of women's bodies as a source of hESC. Especially in relation to these broader concerns, the chapter identifies significant problems relating to the governance of hESC research, and concludes that better deliberative democracy models are needed to address deficits in current debates.

Chapter 3 provides an overview of biobanks and databases, with a case study focus on the UK Biobank, instigated by the Wellcome Trust, which has a primary 'medical' (health) focus; and the UK police national DNA database (NDNAD) which has a primary 'non-medical' goal of tackling crime. The chapter gives an overview of some of the many publics who are engaging with biobanks and databases in the public sphere, identifying the key ways in which they frame, set the stakes of, the debate, such as future-orientated altruism or crime prevention. Because biobanks are a means to an end, publics are often commenting on the actual and potential *end use(s)* or goal(s), and associated risks and benefits, of the bio banks and databases – for example disease cures, treatments and prevention; stigma and discrimination – as much as they comment on the terms (means) of the biobank/database itself, such as how samples are stored and used and in what circumstances. The chapter identifies significant 'governance gaps' particularly in relation to informed consent, benefit-sharing and discrimination. Genetic predictability with regard to common complex disease is shown to be uncertain and highly contested territory with significant implications for health policy, not least concerns about the potential for over-individualised, 'geneticised' responsibility for one's health.

Chapter 4 defines 'pharmacoG' (a combined term for both pharmacogenomics and pharmocogenetics), providing a narrative of the science and the associated products and promises. 'PharmacoG' is defined as a 'hybrid' techno-science involving many different publics including assemblages of governance, science and industry. The chapter then focuses on the concept of the 'bio-economy', namely the economic framework within which pharmacoG is evolving. While some prime movers such as patient groups are happy to support 'big pharma' in their quest for pharmacoG-related cures, others are voicing concerns over issues such as access, ownership (intellectual property) and identity. Much promissory discourse accruing to 'personalised pharmaco' relates to the identification of tiny variations in genetic, genomic and proteomic expression within an individual. The promise of these products is a source of great hope for many patient groups, their advocates, and members of 'disease communities'. However according to others, there are reasons to be critical about how the products (or the idea of them) and specifically targeted potential consumers of these products, are part of the driving economic forces that are shaping this hybrid medical science/industry area, and the implications for public health goals. The chapter identifies narratives of concern around the targeting of specific publics as consumers of potential bio-products.

Chapter 5 focuses on genetic screening and testing, and examines the complex relationship between genetic information and disease knowledge, showing how different publics are negotiating this terrain. The range of available genetic tests in multiple contexts, from prenatal to adult testing, is rapidly widening. The chapter provides an overview of genetic screening and testing practice and policy, using evidence of single-gene disorders. The chapter then focuses on two case study examples of genetic testing; prenatal testing and commercially available adult testing, both of which were catalysing significant public engagement during the research timeframe. This section addresses some of the emergent issues and the ways in which they are being framed by different publics, such as choice, value and 'slippery slopes' in relation to prenatal testing; while commercially available genetic tests raise issues such as how consumers will negotiate risk and what it is they are being sold, returning to the issue of commercially driven patient/consumer identities discussed in the previous chapter.

The increase of genetic testing within public healthcare, and in the availability of commercially available genetic/genomic test kits make this one of the most important arenas of public engagement with human genetics, where many debates about the meanings and implications of genetic information are being situated. The chapter shows that these tests raise complex ethical minefields which must be negotiated. Some see this as the (eugenic) 'slippery slope'; others frame tests in relation to a right to choose on the basis of new information. The efficacy of the use of 'choice' as the key means to frame the debates is questioned. For many, genetic testing and screening informs debates on health and identity, human value and human nature, and social justice and equity. The accuracy of the tests, especially in relation to the predictability of multifactoral disease and assessing predisposition and at-risk status, is also a heavily contested arena.

The final three chapters of this book address in more detail some of the issues and concepts which have been shown in the previous chapters to underpin much public discourse on human genetics. Chapter 6 examines the concept of geneticisation, showing how people construct, and engage with, geneticised accounts of (especially) health and identity in different contexts. A key frame in much genetics discourse is the assumption, implicit or explicit, that there is something 'exceptional' or special about genetic/genomic knowledge, and that it takes precedence over other explanations or knowledge bases. Differentiating between genetic determinism, genetic reductionism and genetic essentialism as different aspects of geneticisation, the chapter first examines the idea that there is something 'exceptional' about genetics providing an overview of genetic exceptionalism and a discussion of where it may and may not have validity as an explanation. There are important policy implications, particularly as an application of genetic exceptionalism is the formation of an ethical imperative to undertake genetic research.

The chapter then focuses on critical public responses to geneticised accounts of health and identity. 'Sustainability citizenship' prime movers, for example, argue that genetic exceptionalism is often overstated and that claims of genetic exceptionalism especially in relation to health often 'frame out' other perspectives such as social justice and poverty alleviation. The assumption of exceptional genetics can operate to exclude or mask other ways of approaching problems, such as social, cultural and economic forces, as well as issues such as inequality. Discourses of genetic exceptionalism are often linked, implicitly or explicitly, to individualist ways of explaining or looking at society. Hence exceptional genetics triggers debates about, and resistance to, notions of individualised responsibility, particularly in relation to health; the chapter examines the implications for citizenship stakes-setting.

Chapter 7 discusses the concepts of choice and consent which have run through accounts of human genetics. Choice and consent are key frames in the donation, or trade, in bio-material such as DNA and human eggs; in debates on genetic testing and screening, for example the use of PGD and PND. They are also central to debates on participation in drugs and biomedical procedures trials and also access to a range of bio-products. Drawing on these examples from previous chapters, this chapter reminds us that these are terms which are constructed, used and also contested by different publics, both in terms of what these 'choices' and 'consents' signify, and in terms of how the concepts themselves measure up as ways of framing the debate. The first half of the chapter examines the use of informed consent in specific circumstances, and shows ways in which it is defined, used, and also challenged, by different prime movers.

The second half of the chapter provides situated examples of how, when, why, where and by whom 'individual choice' is used, responded to and challenged. 'Choice' is consciously used as a key means of framing debates for specific prime movers, notably 'pro research' patient groups and 'pro science' lobby groups. There are important parallels between the discussion about individualised responsibility for one's own health and the idea of an 'individual right to choose'. The implications of such individualised citizenship stakes are identified.

The chapter thus provides specific examples of the limits or problems with the use of choice and consent as tools to frame complex and ambivalent debates. These terms can 'frame out' other important perspectives or mean that they are not easily heard. Informed consent, for example, developed for a specific medical practice, is argued to be too narrow and misses the 'bigger picture' necessary for proper informed consent in contexts such as egg dona-tion. Especially in sensitive and complex arenas such as reproduction and genetics, better forms of participatory democracy are essential to break out of the polarised debate framed in terms of people being 'pro or anti' individual choice or informed consent in specific contexts. It is important to set the debates on some different tracks; to broaden, or to tilt, the frame.

Finally, chapter 8 discusses 'futures talk'. The invocation of the future permeates genetics/genomics discourse; key futures talk can be summarised as 'future promise' (Brown and Michael 2003) and 'future risk'. Importantly, both are contested future territory; what counts as a risk, or a benefit? Values are normative, and hence accounts of future benefits associated with specific applications and techniques are more contested than might at first appear. One person's risk is another's benefit; the enhanced post-human, for example. Situated examples are provided in relation to key types of futures talk under the sub-headings of prediction and uncertainty, risk, 'future promise' and utopias and dystopias. Other framings of the future such as progress, hope and hype are also discussed as sub-sets of 'future promise'.

The chapter argues that the invoked future in genetics discourse is founded on a projection of the present, based both on the values people (individuals, groups, institutions, cultures, societies) hold, and their socio-political and economic predictions, assessments and imperatives about where 'the science' will, might or should go. Thus future predictions are based on competing accounts of current worldviews, and can be seen as a means of persuasion about why specific courses of action should or shouldn't be followed. The meanings people give to genetics in the here and now (not least, the credence they give to the viability of the vaunted science) influence the way in which they invoke the future. Further, specific invocations of the future catalyse public responses; people respond to perceived threats and opportunities inherent in the 'futures talk' of others. There are identifiable hierarchies of power and also of interest; certain groups, political systems and economic pressures are framing the future along a specific axis; uneven power relations are framing specific futures. The chapter concludes that the future promise of cures and treatments in particular has a tendency to drown out other con-cerns, such as risk. Such futures talk thus has profound health and social policy implications; the discourse itself is performing the future into being.

What is 'human genetics'?

'Human genetics' is not a specific thing; it is a diffuse and complex mixture of scientific and technological procedures and applications. A range of social actors are making different knowledge claims about 'human genetics' (Harcourt 2008). Terminology is contested territory and is also shifting exceptionally rapidly as techno-scientific techniques develop and leapfrog over each other. The timeframe covered by this book saw 'the genomics turn'; the use of the term genomics began to overwrite genetics in much scientific and subsequently social science discourse. This was partially a response to the rapid advances in the field of sequencing, causing a shift of scientific focus from the gene to the genome (chapter 4). A Ph.D.'s worth of genetic sequencing ten years ago can now be done in a single afternoon. The transcribing of genetic information is now so fast, scientific prime movers say, that the science of genetics is moving from being able to sequence specific genes, to 'mapping' the genomes of entire species (see chapter 4). Hence 'the genomics turn', the identifiable social performance of genomics discourse (talk), moving out of the lab and into the social sphere. Like genetics, genomics as science performed as social reality is thus impacting on the social world, on issues which matter enormously to people, such as their health, identity, the budgetary spend of nation states and so on.

From a social science perspective, however, there are several concerns with the rather fashionable development of the 'genomics turn' in social discourse, starting with the way language performs a scientific certainty into being. The use of the very conclusive-sounding term 'mapping' is an important example; in fact, genomic 'mapping' is neither scientifically conclusive, nor definitive. There are many information/knowledge gaps, such as the roles of 'junk' and mitochondrial DNA. Further, individual (phenotypical) human genetic expression being variable, there is in fact no such thing as '*the* human genome'. Thus 'the human genome' is not, in essence, definitively mapped at all. 'Mapping' metaphors link easily to promissory discourses, especially from 'big pharma', about how, for example, sequencing one's personalised genomic expression will enable 'a new generation of personalised medicine'. The (contested) significance of these issues in terms of drugs, tests, consumer behaviour, economic capacity and so on are addressed at many different places within the book; for example, see chapters 4, 6 and 8. The development of the field of proteomics, and of Converging Technologies (CT), is set to re-frame the terms of the debate once again. 'Bioscience' could be a useful catch all term for future debates. In an arena of science where disciplinary boundaries are blurring out of all recognition, many are remarking on this confusion of shifting terms and terminologies. In the period 2003–7, CT emerged as an important reality in relation to 'human genetics', as remarked upon by an interviewee in 2004:

> if you go ten, fifteen years in the future, you're not going to be able to distinguish between what's nano technology, what's bio technology, what's information technology or what's genetic engineering. They're all going to be the same kind of technologies … just employed in different ways and different places.

> ('Mike')

In fact, by January 2008 CT in the form of synthetic biology were hitting the headlines (BBC 2008a). The implications of CT generally fall outside the remit of this book, except to identify that they have been the focus of public debate and public action for some time, for example around the environmental risks of nanotechnology (Royal Society 2004; Plows and Reinsborough 2008). Thus it is quite possible that some of the science this book describes will quickly 'go out of date'; for example, developments in synthetic biology, proteomics and Converging Technologies could soon make much of the 'human genetics' science described in this book obsolete. In a fast changing field this is simply inevitable. However, the science described in the book is likely to remain contemporary for several years. Many 'scientific developments' and the issues these raise, described in the book, are at the R&D stage and/or only just starting to impact onto the public sphere. Things move more slowly in techno-science than they appear to – there is a significant difference between discourses of 'future promise' and what actually manifests from out of the lab as a tangible application. Also, the book is a sociological snapshot; it is describing a social phenomenon in a specific space and time, identifying that tomorrow's science, the debates accruing around it, and ultimately social reality are framed, shaped, by previous debates.

CT is an important example of how difficult it is to nail down terms, functions, meanings, in this sphere, or to say where 'wet bench' science leaves off, and technological applications begin. As Andreas Woyke says in relation to nanotechnology,

> The seemingly sharp boundaries between pure and applied research are blurred more than ever before. This point raises the question whether we can legitimately distinguish ... between science and technology.
>
> (Woyke 2008: 14)

The same is true of 'human genetics'; human genetics is 'techno-science' (Haraway 1991), a 'hybrid' site (Latour 1993) where research process and end product blur. For example, stem cell research is described by many in terms of a potential end product and as a research site; and it does indeed exist as both. Diagnostics is both a technological process, and an end product.

Thus genetic/genomic information – 'the science' – associated (potential, actual) applications and a set of narratives about how these will be applied and what they signify, can often be the issue trigger for catalysing social debate and mobilisation, but this is not to put 'the science first'. Science and Technology Studies (STS) literature (Knorr-Cetina 1999; Latour and Woolgar 1979; Latour 1993; Haraway 1991), has established that 'the science' ('techno-science') as a knowledge claim at a specific site, an identifiable thing – 'the gene', for example, 'the human genome' – is identifiably the product, and the reproduction of, social agency, power relations and so on. Because of these multiple influences, these 'hybrid' products are subject to interpretation; they are plural signifiers, not just in terms of multidisciplinary science, but where science, politics and culture blur; they are 'boundary objects' (Star and Griesemer 1989), meaning different things to different people in different contexts. As Woyke says,

> Many subjects and objects of modern science like 'the ozone hole' ... 'the cancer mouse' ... cannot be ... simply or clearly assigned to one or another area of science, for example, cultural, natural, or technological sciences. Partly because they count as at least anthropogenic influenced, and partly because they ... are connected with many very different implications for nature, technology, and culture.
>
> (Woyke 2008: 22)

Scientific and other knowledge claims and associated power relationships frame or shape the thing itself, including how it is named and what these names signify. For example, the term 'junk' DNA is a classic example of how the meaning of the science itself shifts; 'junk' DNA turns out not to be so 'junk' after all.[3] The science is funded, and specific projects and approaches are funded over others; this too shapes the pace and direction of science and technology. Technological applications specifically are very much the direct result of social, economic and political forces. Science is 'nested' within a web of social networks, and the story of the human genetics technologies and associated public engagement given in this book provides further discussion on what some have called the 'politics of technology' (Plows and Reinsborough 2008), particularly in relation to the role of the 'bio-economy' in setting the pace and direction of bio-science (Birch 2006). These issues were key frames for several of the case study 'prime movers', such as the international technology watchdog ETC group, who had a UK-based office during the research timeframe.

Contested definitions of knowledge and expertise arose in relation to public engagement with science and technology during previous environmental and other controversies, such as nuclear power, climate change and GM crops (Bauer 1995; Wynne 1996, 2006; Fischer 2000; Welsh 2000; Purdue 2000; Horlick-Jones, Walls, Rowe *et al.* 2007). These tensions have included calls for a broader debate on what science is 'for', and as such link back to the debates on what public engagement is, and what it is for. There have been disputes about who has the right, and who has the power, to set the terms of the debate in the first place (Grove-White *et al.* 2000; Horlick-Jones, Walls, Rowe *et al.* 2007; Wynne 2006). These critiques are often heard most stridently from the grassroots groups framing challenges to the specific issue at stake (Mayer 2002; Plows and Boddington 2006; Welsh *et al.* 2007).

Much STS work has identified 'the public' right to be taken seriously on questions of scientific knowledge, especially following Wynne's (1996) identification of the 'deficit model' in policy. Wynne identified that much policy assumed that publics opposed science and technological developments because they didn't understand them; that their reactions were the result of a deficit of understanding. Wynne's critique of the 'deficit model' showed how publics have scientific or comparable expertise, using a case study of sheep farmers whose knowledge on the issue of sheep grazing outstripped that of government experts. STS academics have regularly confirmed Wynne's view, that critical and/or oppositional publics are not ones which have deficits in understanding: quite the reverse, as Midden *et al.* (2003) state:

> 'Informedness' has a direct negative effect upon general attitudes, suggesting the more information the public has about biotechnology, the more critical its attitudes will tend to be.
>
> (Midden *et al.* 2003: 214–15)

It is important to note that prime movers' and early risers' propensity to have specific forms of 'expert knowledge', is likely to be different to that of 'the public per se' (Evans and Plows 2007). Academic research has identified patient groups who have 'embodied' expertise about their own conditions (Kerr *et al.* 1998a, b)[4] and patient and other campaign groups who develop scientific expertise. The existence of prime movers with acquired scientific expertise is an important finding of the research project on which this book is based. The NGO GeneWatch, for example, has well established expertise in relation to the science of genetics, and in part, frames its criticisms in scientific terms.

What is seen as relevant or useful knowledge, and thus as relevant expertise, is however a contested subject. Is it 'the science' that one necessarily needs to be an expert in, to discuss concepts of health and equity? In public debates on human genetics, knowledge is often defined in terms of scientific knowledge; bioscientific knowledge has been made to stand in for a range of other knowledge claims. Many people are consistently mixing up talking about 'the science' with talking about the meanings and implications of 'the science'. Other perspectives, such as social justice approaches to health, also contribute important knowledge stakes to 'human genetics' debates which are really 'about' issues of health and identity. Identifying the need to situate discussions of knowledge and expertise more broadly, Jasanoff (2005b) discusses concepts of 'epistemic citizenship' – citizens constructing and contesting meanings, accruing from different knowledge bases and claims. Similarly Harcourt (2008) discusses how different knowledge bases and knowledge claims, are converging in bioscience debates.

Thus what makes the debates about human genetics so difficult to unravel is not only identifying that such debates are often 'about' a range of other things (values, concepts) but also that these other values are themselves sites of contestation, that can be defined and achieved differently through multiple knowledge claims and 'lifeworlds'. These concepts include justice, citizenship, choice, progress, risk, innovation, enhancement, 'human nature', 'the public good' and so on. Often, publics are mobilising because they identify human genetics as supporting or threatening their 'lifeworlds', their values, their claims to knowledge; for example as expressed in discourses about identity, risk or hope. Thus these themes – health, identity, justice, and so on – and what we mean when we use them, what others mean when they use them, are intrinsic to what debates on human genetics are actually *about* for different publics, and are shown to recur consistently across different instances which focus on specific sites of human genetics as a technological application (genetic screening, for example).

These are 'bigger picture' themes in public discourse ostensibly about a specific application of 'human genetics'. The book bridges disciplines to enable more holistic analyses of what publics are doing and saying and why, in relation to human genetics, in particular by synthesising work in sociology of health and medicine concerned with the human body (Rose 2001; Rose 1997; Rabinow 1996; Rose and Novas 2004) with environmental politics approaches to health and identity, environmental social justice and public engagement (Di Chiro 2007, 2008; Epstein 2007), identifying that biologically informed notions of health and identity must take account of environmental social justice issues (Plows and Boddington 2006; Di Chiro 2008). Waldby's (2002) concept of 'bio value' highlights the links between issues of political economy and bioethics, the values people hold, the value(s) they place on things.

Linked closely with the challenging of specific forms of knowledge is the controversy over who counts as an 'expert'; again, an important arena for STS scholars (see Fischer 2000; Irwin 1995; Irwin and Michael 2003; Wynne 2006; Kerr *et al* 1998b; Collins and Evans 2002; Evans and Plows 2007; Plows and Boddington 2006). Challenging the discursive legitimacy of certain types of knowledge, and certain types of expertise, has also formed a core mobilising frame for some of the case study 'prime movers' who have felt that they struggle with 'feeling that we weren't experts, we had no right to speak on the issue, that they would always beat our arguments' ('Dan').

Such concerns about blurring expertise stakes are not confined to the lobby and campaign groups who tend to raise concerns and criticisms, who feel they are 'framed out' of the debates, especially in the media and in policy spheres. A patient group spokesperson made pointed reference to the problem of what constitutes relevant expertise:

> a very senior scientist [was saying] that we would be designing babies in the future ... it was a social prediction ... I'm not convinced that those scientists have the expertise to make such social predictions
>
> ('Peter')

What is seen as relevant knowledge, expertise and who is seen as a relevant stakeholder are thus intrinsically related to how debates are framed, and who has the power to frame them in the public sphere.

Conclusion

Based on qualitative research amongst UK publics during 2003–7, the book examines how specific publics are engaging with human genetics in specific circumstances, how they are framing the stakes of the debates, and what this signifies. Narratives of network relationships between hybrid publics engaging with hybrid techno-science are key to an understanding of public engagement as 'social movement'. In distinguishing between public engagement as policy practice and public engagement as 'social movement' the book is posing the question: 'what is public engagement and what is it *for*?' This chapter has introduced the idea that genetics is constantly being framed in specific ways; such as in the media, in policy consultations, by specific publics, by vested interest. Consequently, many 'prime movers' are interrogating the power relations which enable the framing of human genetics to emerge in a certain way in the public sphere. A recurring theme is the extent to which public groups are responding not only to the specific issues at stake, but also to how the science is governed and how it emerges into the public sphere. People are identifiably making sense of human genetics in terms of their existing experiences, values and knowledge claims – their 'lifeworlds' – especially in relation to issues of health, identity and social justice. The book will show that many 'prime movers' are, or have become, identifiably expert not only in the science, but in relation to the key issues they see as related to the science (Evans and Plows 2007).

Ethnography as a research method is argued to be an important form of 'upstream public engagement', because it can identify emergent, plural, ambivalent accounts in messy social fields. It can also contribute to answering important 'baseline' questions: what are the emergent issues for publics in relation to human genetics? Which publics are mobilising and why? The next chapter introduces the 'cast list' of key players who appear throughout the book. Each subsequent chapter, focusing on a specific genetic site which has been the focus for public engagement, such as biobanking, or a key concept informing this engagement, such as 'geneticisation', provides situated examples of how and why people are debating human genetics, and under what circumstances. It is important to re-emphasise that this is a highly complex social field, and the book simply offers a broad overview of this field, supplemented with some in-depth case study examples. However, the book does aim to cover most of the key issues which were catalysing public engagement in the UK during 2003–7, and provide the resources for further reading, such as policy sites, patient group and watchdog websites, and so on. Some issues and examples are covered in greater detail, and appear more 'in the spotlight' than others. For example, the HFEA's policy moves in 2006 over the use of women's eggs is covered in detail, but other HFEA policy moves are not. The book does not aim to be definitive in the account it gives of public groups and their key frames; it simply aims to provide some more detailed ethnographic examples of 'public engagement', identifying that there are multiple sites and ways in which publics are engaging. It is to these publics which we now turn in chapter 1.

1 Methodology and publics overview

Introduction

First, this chapter further interrogates what is meant by 'public engagement', showing how social movement theory (SMT) tools and principles have informed both a definition of public engagement with human genetics, and the accompanying methodology for studying it. Hybrid, fluid publics are shown to be engaging with human genetics in many different contexts. This first section also defines, and provides examples of, the sorts of public engagement identified during the research. Second, the chapter discusses the qualitative methods which formed the basis for data collection. Third, this chapter introduces a 'cast list' of the different publics whose voices are heard throughout the book. This section introduces the two case study sites which were the core focus of qualitative research; environmental social justice and Disability Rights groups who for various reasons tend to be cautious about or critical of human genetics applications; and patient groups and their supporters, who tend to be extremely supportive of them. This section also introduces other civil society groups who are engaging in the debates, noting that scientists, policy makers and the media are also key 'prime movers'. An overview of 'the general public' and how 'the general public' engages, or could engage, with human genetics provides further reflections on concepts of hybrid civil society.

Section one: researching public engagement with human genetics

A social movement theory (SMT) approach was undertaken for the identification, understanding and theorising of public engagement with human genetic technologies. Whilst a 'social movement' is a specific type of collective protest behaviour,[1] SMT concepts can be seen as tools in a toolbox, used to understand a range of types of public engagement/social life (Doherty *et al.* 2003). One of the most straightforward uses of SMT informing this book is the description of social interaction as interaction between networks. Much public engagement with genetics can be described as the interaction of and between social networks of various types, in very different settings. Social movements – and other sorts of social networks – operate through fluid network activity, disseminating information, constructing identities, and developing sets of meanings, or frames (Diani 1992). These interactive, organic, horizontal (that is, non-hierarchical) network processes have been defined as 'rhizomic' (Deleuze and Guattari 1987). Resources such as information and knowledge (values, meanings) are disseminated between networks with 'weak ties' links to each other (Granovetter 1973; Carroll and Ratner 1996). Understanding public engagement with human genetics in terms of the network relationships which individuals and groups have with each other enables an understanding of social hybridity and assemblage as the links people make when catalysed by specific issues and circumstances.

Informed by social movement theory, 'public engagement' is defined in this book as a self-starting social phenomenon – *social movement* – as well as being a specific form of policy process. Public engagement is thus defined as the phenomenon and process of multiple publics engaging with human genetics in multiple ways, including protest activity. For example, a Disability Rights protest about prenatal genetic screening for Down's syndrome is public engagement. A radio phone-in on 'saviour siblings' is public engagement. Scientists being interviewed in the media about 'breakthroughs' is public engagement. Public engagement of this type represents much of the data on which this book is based.

Another important term is mobilisation. Tarrow (1998) discusses mobilisation as social movement activity; mobilisation is both the process, and the end result, of activist networks. The terms mobilisation, and mobilising publics, are used throughout the book to emphasise the sense of public engagement as an active phenomenon, consciously undertaken by different social actors; people engage, people mobilise, over human genetics, in many different ways. The introduction discussed the importance of the concepts of 'prime movers' (McAdam 1986), and 'early risers' (Tarrow 1998), in the mobilisation process. Framing, an important social movement concept, was outlined in the introduction as being central to an understanding of how different actors develop their worldviews, or 'lifeworlds' (Habermas 1987) in specific contexts. Most of the actors described in the book are prime movers and early risers, many of whom were predisposed to mobilise, because their groups and networks predated 'human genetics' as an emergent social phenomenon. These groups thus brought their pre-existing frames to the 'human genetics' debates, and developed these frames in this new context (Nelkin 1995; Plows and Reinsborough 2008). Melucci (1996) describes how social movements go through periods of dormancy or 'latency', and that out of such latent networks prime movers and early risers emerge to frame the stakes of the debates, and to catalyse mobilisation.

The social geographer Paul Routledge has written about the ways in which specific social networks create 'convergence spaces' (Routledge 1996, 2003). The term convergence space can be taken to mean the conscious creation of (generally, but not exclusively) physical space by specific people (groups, networks) who then converge, within or through it. Such convergence spaces can catalyse hybrid activity. Thus broadly defined, a convergence space can consist of anything; a typical example would be a workshop, or a prearranged online blog session between geographically dispersed social actors. A protest can be seen as a convergence space. A meeting of the UK Human Genetics Commission (HGC) can be seen as a convergence space. 'Accidental' or 'organic' convergence spaces can occur; an informal meet-up of scientists around the water cooler can be a convergence space. A patient group 'prime mover' making fortuitous hyperlinks online creates a convergence space. Throughout the book, situated examples are given of the sorts of public engagement techniques which different publics employ. The key forms of this mobilisation can be summarised as being:

- networking (informal and formal) and capacity building within groups and networks
- protests
- lobbying
- input into policy/regulatory processes
- public education, 'awareness raising' and engagement work; events, literature, websites
- constructing, and interacting with, others as 'allies or enemies'

Different chapters provide specific examples of this broad range of public engagement. For example, campaign groups often run workshop events consciously aimed at capacity building primarily within their own existing networks and groups. An example is the workshops on genetics, science and technology at the European Social Forum (ESF) in London, 2004 (Welsh *et al.* 2007). The ESF is an annual event of European grassroots networks, groups, NGOs and far-left political parties, and is an important event in the constantly co-constructed process of global civil society networks which have been termed the 'anti' [alter] globalisation movement. Whilst high-visibility 'summit hopping' by 'the movement of movements' at G8 and similar summits is part of a now long established repertoire of action[2], events like the ESF show the more latent work of movement capacity building. Participant observation was conducted at this event, which involved participating in the workshops being run on human genetics and bioscience more generally. Appendix 3 is a list of these workshops. It shows what human genetics developments/applications were catalysing mobilisation at the time, how these were framed, and which groups and networks were 'prime movers' and 'early risers'. These are very much emergent frames and show the process of meaning construction in action. Generally, groups and individuals within these sorts of networks are often predisposed to undertake protest activity, which often performs a symbolic function and not always (or just) a disruptive one. Importantly, some of these groups will also engage with policy processes. Campaign groups and networks, especially the more 'established' charities and NGOs, also have a strong focus on 'awareness raising', for example through websites, publications and public events. These are the more public-facing aspect of network and group and NGO activity, for example the publications produced by the UK NGO/'watchdog' GeneWatch and the patient charity AMRC in relation to issues such as genetic testing. Many of the groups which engage in this way also engage with policy and regulation as 'expert stakeholders', for example responding to public consultations.

Public engagement defined as a policy practice, and 'public consultation' as a specific form of policy-defined public engagement, are very different types of public engagement, and are the primary means by which policy engages with public opinion. Public engagement as policy 'best practice' was developing in scope in the research timeframe. In Brussels in 2005 the EU held a forum entitled 'Science in Society'[3] which fed back the results of EU-wide policy initiatives to develop means of engaging with different publics and identifying their views; this is part of ongoing EU policy to develop public engagement as an integrated part of informing science policy through widening the stakes for future initiatives. A UK-led initiative which actively fed into the Science in Society event was the concept of 'upstream public engagement' (Wynne 2006; Wilsden and Willis 2004) which aims to engage 'key stakeholders' earlier on in the planning processes to better identify risks and benefits. Other recent policy-orientated initiatives which aim to develop public engagement methods and outputs include citizens juries (Greenpeace 2005) and 'science cafés'.[4]

However despite such laudable aims, which have certainly improved public engagement approaches, public engagement as policy practice is still strongly criticised by many different participants. Many 'prime movers' identify limited terms and remits, and hence end results, embedded within policy-led public engagement, especially public consultations. These limits are even acknowledged by policy makers. The 'Effective Consultation' Cabinet Office report cited in the introduction identified public cynicism, even – or especially – amongst those who already engage in such processes, who asked the rhetorical question: what is the point of engagement? For a policy process to be underway, someone, somewhere has already set the stakes, and thus identified who counts as a stakeholder. There is much criticism, sometimes acknowledged by policy and regulatory authorities, of how agendas are being set in relation to human genetics and science generally; certain groups feel there is a lack of legitimacy for certain frames, whilst other accounts are privileged. From this perspective, even 'upstream' public engagement, which aims to include identified stakeholders early on in consultation processes, can be seen as having limited use when the policy agenda (and hence the identification of stakes, and stakeholders) has itself been set so far 'upstream' by politically powerful actors. The ensuing public debates have been 'framed' on many counts; publics thus have no option but to respond to issues as they emerge on terms they would not necessarily have set themselves. Many prime movers and other publics are wary of public engagement, and whilst they might engage with the processes, they usually have quite cynical expectations about what this may achieve. Because of this, they choose to develop their own forms of engagement including forms of protest (Welsh *et al.* 2007) in order to set their own agendas on their own terms. How the stakes of public engagement are set, and how different groups struggle to re-frame the stakes of the debate, are key issues in this book and are returned to in different settings.

Science communication can be seen as a form of public engagement. The rise of science communication as an actual academic discipline is significant. Imperial College launched the first science communication masters degree in the UK in 1991 (and also supervises doctoral students), citing these opportunities as 'highly relevant to those seeking careers in public engagement or science policy'.[5] Resources have been invested, from both public and private funding sources, to promote 'public communication of science'. The Science Museum's Dana Centre, for example, 'takes a fresh, no-holds-barred look at the biggest issues in science today'.[6] This has laudable aims – it is essential to make science accessible – but there is also a danger that such approaches rely on a 'deficit model' of public understanding of science. Several science departments and projects are running philosophy and social science programmes in parallel with their work on human genetics, such as University College, London (UCL ca. 2008). What is significant here, is the acknowledgement from the natural science 'prime movers' running such courses, that other disciplines, perspectives, 'lifeworlds', have much to offer the natural sciences in terms of identifying what the key issues at stake are; in framing the debates in a different way. Bucchi (2004) identifies 'cross-talk' between scientists and publics. This 'cross-talk' has the potential to 'tilt the frame' through an open approach to issues of meaning, knowledge and expertise in relation to human genetics debates. It has the potential to feed back to policy in terms of identifying a broader range of stakes and stakeholders.

Section two: methodology

The data used in this book was drawn from a three-year UK academic project on public engagement with human genetic technologies, entitled 'The Emerging Politics of Human Genetic Technologies',[7] undertaken between 2003 and 2006/7.[8] The predominant focus was on the UK, with attention also paid to EU and international publics, where the data was available within the limited scale of the project. The social dynamics of multiple publics were traced, identifying core areas of interest and concern in relation to a broad variety of issues and themes. This process first identified those social actors who were a very visible presence on the social stage. Informed by previous research by the research team (Chesters and Welsh 2006; Plows 2003, 2004; Doherty *et al.* 2003, 2007), the project also identified social networks, groups and individuals who were predisposed to become engaged in the debates, or whose existing frames and forms of engagement were arguably less well represented in consultation processes and in other policy/public settings than some more visible others. Identifying these more hidden voices enabled an overview of a broader pool of social actors, and it is the potential of this data to inform and develop the debates on 'human genetics' which is a key focus in this book.

The research methodology was qualitative, drawing first on documentary and other types of data logged at specific sites and events, including online data such as web blogs and websites, noting an increasing tendency for people located in specific places to use the internet, for example by ordering genetic tests online. A key qualitative method used was ethnography or participant observation, which is a means of understanding a social phenomenon through personal participation in events by the researcher. Participant observation was deliberately developed as a methodological form of 'upstream public engagement' in that participation in grassroots settings enabled a clear view of what people were doing and saying in relation to human genetics *on their own terms* (Plows 2008a). Such participant observation is founded on principles of 'grounded theory' (Hammersley 1993) in that it was inductive; the project was led by what was discovered in grassroots settings, in interviews and in different public settings such as media debates. Importantly, through this use of participant observation, public engagement was thus traced opportunistically as it emerged onto the social stage in response to specific events such as specific policy moves. Early signs were picked up of emergent public controversies which have now 'broken', such as the creation of hybrid embryos (chapter 2), not to mention issues which could potentially become major public controversies, such as the unregulated use of nanoparticles in a range of goods (Plows and Reinsborough 2008). Other examples include the range of responses in relation to the sourcing and proposed use of women's eggs for biomedical research (Plows 2007b, 2008b); (chapter 2), and social responses in relation to the police DNA database (chapter 3).

Participant observation thus enabled a broad range of public engagement events, both self-initiated by civil society groups (such as workshops and protest events), and those initiated by policy processes, such as public consultation exercises, to be identified in the timeframe. The use of qualitative methods in an exceptionally diverse, multifaceted and 'messy' (Law 2006) research field, necessitated taking snapshots to get a sense of this field. The research goal was not to map out a comprehensive overview, which would have been encyclopaedic in scale, but rather it aimed to get a workable sense of the bigger picture, through these snapshots and soil samples; for example of what types of genetics applications were causing social engagement; what sorts of policy and regulatory bodies were dealing with the issues. The research did focus, however, on establishing a more comprehensive overview of the range of civil society groups and organisations who were identified as engaging with human genetics during the project's timeframe. In particular, as discussed in Section three of this chapter, qualitative methods were used to elicit the views and forms of engagement used by networks in two case study sites; environmental social justice activists and patient groups. However, for example, no specific ethnography was done with patient groups identified with genetic conditions and the interactions which ensue between these individuals, other family members, and genetic counsellors and other medical practitioners, although reference is made to relevant research (chapter 5). Thus this is not a definitive account of public engagement with genetics as it developed within the timeframe of the research, and this is an important methodological qualifier.

Further, a number of interviews with 'prime movers' were conducted, to get a more in-depth sense of what sorts of issues these individuals were engaging with, how they framed those issues, and how they then engaged with them and with whom. Interviewees were identified using a 'snowball' technique and through the process of ethnographic research. The interviews were particularly useful for in-depth accounts from highly knowledgeable, 'expert' publics, and for identifying complexity and ambivalence – 'beyond pro and anti' – in their perspectives. A list of the interviewees whose narratives are drawn on in this book is given in Appendix 1.

Section three: 'cast list' of publics

An introductory cast list of other important publics, many of them early risers and prime movers, identified during the project is given below. Even in the primary case study site, the book gives only a glimpse of this complex picture, providing some examples of the complex typologies and relationships which exist between actors in these social networks. Different chapters introduce specific narratives of publics across scientific, regulatory and civil society spheres, mobilising in relation to specific issues, and/or specific techniques; for example, stem cell research or pharmacogenetics. These contextualised examples show how different publics form hybrid assemblages, and draw lines, in relation to specific issues.

Case study 1: 'sustainability citizenship' networks

The networks and groups in this case study are broadly and loosely connected through what have elsewhere been described by the author as 'sustainability citizenship' approaches to human genetics (Plows and Boddington 2006). 'Sustainability citizenship' (Barry 2005) is defined as a politicised focus on social and environmental justice and equity, including access to decision-making mechanisms, identifying imbalances in power relations and the role of political economy in setting aims and agendas. In relation to human genetics, some have referred to an overarching framework of the 'politics of technology': 'what we need to get to is ... the politics of new technologies ... how new technologies impact on society, how society has some control over that'('Mike').

A similar analysis was expressed in a 'Green Action' (2004) briefing for environmentally-focused activists:

Technology is political. Social forces shape technology ... technology ... becomes a social force that in return shapes society ... The desires and interests (or ignorances) of those who control the design process are what shape technology.[9]

If there are politics of technology there are also cultures of technology attached to them. People's values are reflected and re-framed and refracted through the sorts of technologies available to them; and those technologies have a politics, as 'Mike' identifies. The specifics of 'sustainability citizenship' discourses are developed in this book *in situ* in relation to specific contexts, such as human egg sourcing, as actors identify key stakes. Sustainability citizenship is discussed in more detail in chapter 6 as being an important alternative framework to 'geneticised' accounts of health and identity. Broadly, in relation to human genetics, themes of self, identity, health and the body, which have tended to be constructed in terms of individual responsibility, have quickly been picked up and re-framed by such actors in terms of health and its relationship with environmental social justice, social policy provision and global/local citizenship stakes.

The case study focused on a UK-based loose network composed of a variety of different 'prime mover and early riser' groups connected by a broad adherence to sustainability citizenship as defined above. Many of these groups are well established NGOs and campaign groups who are identified as 'key stakeholders' in relevant regulatory frameworks. These include Disability Rights campaigners such as Disability Awareness in Action; health, environmental and social justice NGOs such as The CornerHouse, Corporate Watch, and EcoNexus; civil liberties and consumer rights campaign groups such as Liberty and the Consumers Association; and genetic and technology 'Watchdogs' and NGOs such as Human Genetics Alert, GeneWatch, GM Watch and the influential international watchdog ETC Group, which, during the period under study had a UK-based office. Some of these established NGOs and watchdogs have 'weak ties' with loose, autonomous networks of 'anti-globalisation'[10] and environmental activists; the networks which took direct action over GM crops in the late 1990s (Welsh *et al.* 2007; Routledge 2003; Ainger *et al.* 2003).

The case study 'prime movers' were, in the majority of cases, already mobilising over health, identity, civil liberties, and environmental and social justice issues, and in some cases were already involved in mobilisations where global capitalism has been framed in terms of the adverse impacts this economic framework has had on individuals, communities and the environment. They were therefore predisposed to be engaging with human genetic/genomic genetic science and technologies; these are converging discourses (Plows and Boddington 2006; Welsh *et al.* 2007; Plows and Reinsborough 2008). Some of these are grassroots activists coming from the margins (Harry *et al.* 2000; Howard 2001); such groups, networks and communities are quick to recognise what they see as further threats to their environment, identity and life chances.

The contexts in which these groups and networks come together are multiple. Very importantly, these groups and networks are usually loosely,

informally connected and are characterised by these fluid and organic relationships. Thus the links between these and other groups can vary from strong
alliances in specific contexts – such as over civil liberties issues catalysed by
the police DNA database – to more 'weak ties' links which are made more
informally between groups. Ethnographic trails were traced out to Europe,
Canada and America as individuals and groups made network connections,
catalysed by specific triggers such as policy shifts. Some key international
links include the German feminist network ReproKult, the US-based watchdog Genetics and Society, the Indigenous Peoples Council and the People's
Health Movement. The groups in the case study have further network links
and ties, in structural or in more informal ways, with a multitude of other
groups and individuals, including those among the spheres of governance
(policy and regulatory bodies) and those involved in the production of the
science itself (broadly defined). The NGO GeneWatch, for example, has well
developed network contacts with UK regulatory frameworks who see Gene-
Watch as an 'expert stakeholder' in certain settings; GeneWatch similarly has
an extensive network of contacts within the 'scientific community' and within
academic settings, such as through the ESRC Genomics Network. The book
provides narrative accounts of how in different circumstances, hybridity
occurs between international NGOs, global health bodies such as the World
Health Organisation, UK regulators such as the HGC, with local campaign
groups and so on.

Case study 2: 'pro genetics' patient groups and advocates

Identity is highly contested territory in relation to health, and there are many
different types of, definitions of and ways of constructing, patient groups.
'Patients' as a general term represents a number of different groups, individuals and networks who do not necessarily mobilise by default in favour of
human genetics research. Disability Rights groups, for example, generally
identify broader themes of access to social resources in relation to health
provision, identifying risks as well as benefits in relation to human genetics.
Many people encounter genetics in a medical setting as individuals and do
not get involved with patient campaign group activity; for example, people
who are diagnosed with genetic conditions may not even tell other family
members, or choose to 'keep it within the family'.

However the patient groups in this case study are ones which have tended
to proactively support human genetics and associated bioscience research,
such as stem cell research, and tend to work closely together to further this
agenda through a range of campaign and lobbying techniques. Importantly,
these generally 'pro genetics' groups will also identify risks and concerns, in
specific contexts; this is ambivalent territory. They include Genetic Interest
Group, the patient group Seriously Ill for Medical Research, now called
Patients Voice for Medical Advance, and the Association of Medical
Research Charities. Closely connected in this network cluster are a number of

'pro science' lobby groups; Progress Educational Trust, the Institute of Ideas, and Sense About Science.

A small sample of patient 'prime movers' were interviewed and their views and modes of engagement were also traced through participant observation in a range of public events which such groups participated in, or initiated, such as the Institute of Ideas *Genes and Society* event held in London, 2003, and Progress Educational Trust's 2005 public debate on the police DNA database held in Cardiff. The book provides contextualised examples of how such patient groups and their allies have consistently supported and promoted bioscience research, framing discourses of hope and expectation in relation to the potential for the technologies to cure and treat a range of conditions. These patient groups have close network ties with other medical charitable foundations, with regulatory bodies, with pharmaco industry (popularly described as 'big pharma'), which sponsors activity undertaken by actors in this case study cluster, and with the research scientists themselves. The following provides a useful account of the links between the patient and 'pro science' groups, policy and 'big pharma':

> BioNews is a web- and email-based source of news, information and comment in human genetics and assisted reproduction ... The development of BioNews.org.uk was funded by an educational grant from the Department of Health. BioNews by Email is sponsored by AstraZeneca. Our sponsors have no editorial input into BioNews: full editorial control rests with the publisher, Progress Educational Trust.
>
> (PET 2005)

Many patient groups, whatever their position on specific techno-scientific techniques and research agendas, are highly adept in achieving their aims of attracting high public visibility to campaign for resources and research. A wealth of patients' perspectives are to be found in material produced by patient groups themselves, especially prime mover patient groups who have developed capacity in lobbying, public engagement and campaigning over time. Through the mobilisation process, patient group prime movers develop 'lay' expertise (Wynne 1996; Kerr *et al.* 1998a, b); meaning they can become extremely knowledgeable about specific medical conditions, the science behind them, the relevance of genetic information, the stage of research in terms of treatments and cures and so on; something very evident in 'Susan's account:

> I'd looked up CF [Cystic Fibrosis] from the moment 'Emily' was diagnosed at three and a half months ... I wanted to know all about the condition, all about what was available, all about how research was moving because when you are told that your baby might not see five, you ... look as a parent to everything that's available.
>
> ('Susan')

Patient groups claiming 'embodied expertise' have also both challenged and supported what counts as scientific knowledge (Kerr *et al.* 1998a, b; Tutton *et al.* 2005). The idea of embodied expertise is that someone directly, physically, experiencing a condition has knowledge about it (for example, about what sorts of symptoms are experienced); such knowledge claims are argued as being comparable with scientific and medical knowledge. This has made an extremely important contribution to the understanding of public engagement with medicine, science and technology.

Broader 'cast list' overview

The subsections below provide an introductory overview of other important prime movers engaging with human genetics, including policy and regulatory bodies, scientists, the media and other civil society groups.

Besides the two case study sites, several other civil society campaign or 'interest groups' (Tait 2001) were visibly engaging with human genetics during the timeframe of the research, and situated cast lists and narratives which give issue-specific examples of these groups and networks are provided throughout the book. To take an example, perhaps the most publicly visible civil society group is the pro-life group Comment on Reproductive Ethics (CORE), which has significant expertise in engaging both with the media and the regulatory sphere. CORE has been extremely vocal in opposing uses of human embryos in bioscience research, and in opposing genetics and reproduction generally, for example in terms of prenatal screening. CORE has some interesting 'strange bedfellows' connections with other campaign groups, which are discussed in chapters 2 and 5. Importantly, pro-life perspectives have dominated many debates on human genetics; in this book, more attention has been paid to the case study sustainability citizenship cluster, as a deliberate means of highlighting other voices which are less well heard above pro-life opposition.

'Science' is shaped by social spaces informed by power, politics and economics (Latour and Woolgar 1979; Knorr-Cetina 1999; Birch 2006), and scientists can be seen as social actors within a socially constructed space. Scientists as individuals are located within institutions and operate within interrelated networks, like any other social group. 'Scientists' are a very diverse collection of individuals, networks and organisations; there is massive variation in outlook, remit, power relations and so forth. Scientist narratives in this book are shown to comprise a very varied landscape. A small sample of interviews were conducted with scientists, and this sample was boosted with other forms of qualitative data derived from participant observation and through following specific narratives of events, such as the use of human embryos for stem cell research. Overviews of scientific bodies who are key participants were undertaken. There is a standard list of UK science institutions who are key genetics/genomics players, including funding bodies, such as the Medical Research Council, and the Biotechnology and Biological

Sciences Research Council. Both of these are government funded, and there are also significant charity and private foundations which fund medical and scientific research such as the Wellcome Trust. Bodies such as the Royal Society have a quasi-governance function and often take an advisory role and/or take a public stance on specific issues.

There are specific places where specialised scientific research of various types is carried out, often attached in different ways to different university sites; the Sanger centre, which focuses on genetic, genomic and proteomic sequencing work; stem cell research centres such as the North East England Stem Cell Institute (NESCI), and individual research teams operating on highly specific projects within these institutions such as the Rayner lab at the Sanger Institute.[11] These 'convergence spaces' generate social network activity which can be seen to co-construct scientific practice.

The book provides several examples of the melding between publicly funded and privately funded science, comprising a multitude of different 'hybrid' permutations between, for example, university science and private 'spin out' companies; these are often referred to as Public Private Partnerships (PPPs). Glasner and Rothman (2004) have termed these PPPs 'co-laboratories'. 'Big pharma' are linked into these co-laboratories in a number of ways (chapter 4). The UK government has funded a number of 'GeneParks' whose core function is to facilitate genetic/omic research and help translate university research into applications which will be taken up by private investment. The GeneParks are funded both by the Department of Health and by the Department of Trade and Industry, indicating a merging of a health agenda with an economic agenda which is a consistent narrative in the book:

> how would ... 'UK PLC' ... capitalise, commercialise ... the potential of the human genome sequence? And also how would it be used within the NHS to the benefit of patients? So out of that came this concept of the genetics knowledge park [GenePark] network, to link basic research in genetics, to translate that research.
>
> ('Ian')

There are a vast number of policy and regulatory bodies and institutions, and government departments, which have responsibility for the governance of human genetics research and development (R&D). Some areas of human genetics are extensively regulated and other areas have significant 'governance gaps'. Some of the regulatory bodies and institutions are directly responsible for policy setting and 'quality control', such as the Human Fertilisation and Embryology Authority (HFEA). Government departments are proactively constructing policy on the basis of genetics 'future promise' and 'future risk' (chapter 8) especially in the areas of crime, health and economic development in relation to science and technology. The Department of Health has set long-term policy goals along certain pathways through the promissory discourses accruing to health and genetics framed in its white paper 'Our inheritance, our future' (Dept of Health 2003). The Department for Business Innovation and Skills (who change their name frequently) takes a proactive policy and regulatory line in facilitating economic development of genetics and related bio-research. Other institutions, such as the HGC, have more of an advisory/ public engagement role, but they are still very much part of 'official' regulatory structures.

Specific regulatory bodies have jurisdiction in relation to specific arenas.

> it depends on the types of issues, for example, if we were talking about genetics and employment, we might talk to people from the Health and Safety Executive or the Disability Rights Commission. If we were talking about insurance we might want to talk to people from the Treasury.
>
> ('Angela')

For example, the HFEA is responsible for regulating stem cell research (chapter 2); the Home Office is responsible for the police national DNA database (chapter 3); the National Institute for Clinical Excellence for regulatory oversight relating to pharmaco products (chapter 4); and the Genetics and Insurance Committee and the National Screening Council (NSC) for genetic screening regulation (chapter 5). Multiple regulatory bodies may be involved in the process of monitoring a specific technology through different stages of R&D and application; for example, in setting 'informed consent' standards relating to participation in biomedical research in specific circumstances. Parliament's two Select Committees covering science also have an advisory role in examining government policy,[12] and have reported on several aspects of human genetics such as the regulation of hybrid and chimera embryos (HoC 2007), and genomic medicine (HoL 2009). Other bodies are also linked to the governance process through advisory roles, such as the Nuffield Council on Bioethics.

With a mandate from these regulatory and policy frameworks, the governance sphere is characterised by a proliferation of ethical committees set up to provide, and monitor, 'best practice' guidelines in multiple situations of 'governance gaps' in specific contexts; for example, the recently established UK Biobank Ethics and Governance Council whose job is to set standards relating to the parameters of donating DNA samples to the UK Biobank (chapter 3). Especially in the governance gaps formed as new technologies develop rapidly, the regulatory sphere is characterised by the 'hybrids' which form between the producers of the science and existing regulatory frameworks. The UK Biobank ethics council (chapter 3) and the UK stem cell bank (chapter 2) are important examples of new forms of hybrid governance emerging through the development of new technologies.

Regulatory and policy bodies also interact with different publics. Different bodies and institutions will engage publics at different stages and in different ways. 'Expert stakeholders' are called to give evidence at select committee hearings; other publics can struggle to gain access to these more closed policy frameworks and have to rely on public consultation processes, by which time stakes have already been set. Patient groups and scientists would seem, anecdotally, to have the best access to regulatory frameworks; see the 'bionews' example given above.

Specific UK regulation and policy is discussed *in situ*, for example stem cell research is discussed in chapter 2. As 'Angela' points out, 'the UK position can at times be quite unique ... for example on stem cell research'.

UK policy is made independently of European policy, but there has been a recent EU legal case which impacts directly on UK policy; the recent EU human rights ruling on the storage of DNA samples in specific circumstances on the police national DNA database is discussed in chapter 3. European regulation is thus relevant to the UK, and UK regulatory bodies keep abreast of how the European Commission is addressing bioscience issues. An influential body is the European Group on Ethics in Science and New Technologies which is, in its own words,

> a neutral, independent, pluralist and multidisciplinary body which advises the European Commission on ethical aspects of science and new technologies in connection with the preparation and implementation of Community legislation or policies.
>
> (EGE 2000)

There are also a number of international bodies, some of which are advisory bodies specifically set up to advise on genetics/genomics issues, such as the Human Genome Organisation. Other global institutions, especially those whose remits include governance on health and economic development, have also engaged with human genetics and produced a number of reports, including the World Health Organisation and the Organisation for Economic Co-operation and Development. Trade Related Intellectual Property Rights and patenting rulings, relevant to human genetics, are internationally related through the World Trade Organisation and World Intellectual Property Organization.

'Members of the general public' can potentially mobilise at any time, if catalysed to do so; if they identify with the issues at stake. For example a 'member of the public' may be catalysed to get more involved with a specific campaign group if diagnosed with a genetic condition, or asked if they wish to donate to a DNA biobank. In fact it is the increased, and increasing, impact of genetics/genomics and related bio and reproductive technologies on 'the general public' in specific arenas which means that public engagement will deepen and develop as people see themselves more as stakeholders in what is occurring and wish to take part in the accompanying debates. A further important methodological observation is that if 'human genetics debates' are set in broader terms of citizenship, health and identity, then many more people would immediately identify themselves as stakeholders. Thus there are multiple potential publics who could be constructed as engaged in the debates, depending on how the stakes are set. The project aimed to identify some of these potential voices, again limited by the practicalities of a small qualitative sample.

Snapshots of different public narratives occur in various examples throughout the book. 'The general public' is engaging with human genetics in several ways. They are engaging with specific (media, policy) debates cata-lysed by shifts in science and/or science policy – for example, public responses to 'saviour siblings' in 2005 (chapter 5). They are becoming more directly engaged with human genetics, for example being asked to donate their DNA (chapter 3), or through being diagnosed with a genetic condition (chapter 5). How publics become patients or construct genetic accounts of their identities is an important, emergent, social phenomenon discussed throughout the book. Finally, publics are engaging with human genetics as bio-consumers: they are engaging through the consumption of bio-products such as a genetic test bought online (chapter 5). The book provides examples of the complex blurring between publics, patients and consumers, and seeks to unpack the significance of these blurring identities (chapters 4, 5).

The media contributes significantly to the debates on human genetics; however the media was not the subject of detailed analysis in the project. To redress this balance slightly, the following narrative provides an overview. For examples of dedicated academic media analysis, see Haran *et al.* (2007) and Horlick-Jones, Walls, Kitzinger *et al.* (2007). 'Human genetics' is rarely out of the media, and occasionally 'big stories' break, triggering public debates, often on accompanying public blogs. The media is integral to the conducting of public debates about human genetics, and most mobilising groups try to enlist media attention in a variety of ways, some of them more successful than others, to communicate their point of view. This is the case even when actors are extremely cynical about the media's ability to tell their side of the story. Policy, political and scientific actors all use the media to communicate, and this is often the starting point for the way stories leave the lab or the policy document, and how debates are then framed in the public sphere and the way the public uptakes them: for example, saviour siblings, hybrid embryos.

Those with power and/or an already-established 'public legitimacy' such as a scientist or policy maker can start a media story with far less effort than, say, a struggling campaign group; this is not necessarily the media's 'fault', however, and says more about the reiterative nature of power and culture in contemporary societies. That being said, the tendency of the media to return to the same 'usual suspects' for quotes and soundbites for their news stories can fairly be criticised; issues are framed, and stakes are set, which by default excludes (or makes very difficult) the possibility of re-framing these stakes to ask different questions, and to enrol the perspectives of different stakeholders. Many scientists have become extremely media-savvy and enjoy exceptional media access.

'The media' consists of multiple formats including newspapers, radio, tele-vision and the internet, which increasingly tend to blur together; for example, most UK newspapers also web-mount their content and have a strong web presence. Multiple positions are taken by different newspapers and specific columnists, and there is a great deal of difference between the remit of a science and technology correspondent, and a news desk headline writer. The enrolling of 'the media' as scapegoat for all the woes accruing to the conducting of public debates on human genetics rings a little hollow, given this huge variety in media form, content and approach. A typical example of 'usual suspect' media framing in relation to genetics and bioscience stories is the 'breakthrough'.[13] 'Breakthroughs' are regularly enrolled in media stories, in relation to a new technique, or scientific discovery, which is generally framed – by the media commentator, or the scientific spokesperson concerned – as being potentially able to provide disease and condition treatment or cure. 'Breakthrough' frames change as the science evolves; stem cell 'breakthroughs' (chapter 2) are as common now as 'gene for' breakthrough stories were, for example 'the first bioengineered windpipe utilising the patient's own stem cells' (BBC 2008d, Bristol 2008).

'The media' are often castigated for 'scaremongering' stories, and for polarising complex debates into black or white headlines, for example with 'expert scientists' in one corner, and 'the public' in the other. They are also criticised for a tendency to use the example of an individual, such as a sick child, to provide the 'human face' of a story (chapter 8). Certain patient groups are extremely experienced in using the media as a means of promoting their aims. What concerns others about the use of sick children to promote research 'breakthroughs', is that to voice concerns and caveats (even, say, about scientific validity), makes one appear to be unsympathetic to the fate of the specific child.

Interestingly, groups on all sides castigate the media for 'hype' (chapter 8). Talking about the way media report on medical 'breakthroughs', 'Peter' noted that

> it's a thousand and one tiny improvements. ... that's how medical research really works and. ... the media debate and public debate get almost a little bit ahead of themselves into the controversial areas.
>
> ('Peter')

There is plenty of evidence of 'hype' stories; there will be cures tomorrow; for example, 'Gene therapy offers hope of cure for HIV' (*Independent* (2009) based on G. Hütter *et al.* (2009)). 'Cures tomorrow' stories occur when reportage about potential developments in a specific technique is over-hyped. 'Breakthrough' discourse, for example, often turns out to have little substance behind it: a discovery relating to genetic information, or a development in a technique, is not a cure. 'Horror' stories, for example about 'Frankenstein' hybrid embryos – 'Docs to create mootant cells' (*Sun* 2006) – are also quite common. The media's job is not to be a public service 'for the communication of science'. The media's role is to sell papers and tell stories. Similarly the media's job is not to provide coverage per se for campaign groups across the spectrum. Something which is clearly an issue is not necessarily a newsworthy story. The media's rationale – selling papers, telling stories – is why risk and benefit stories can blur and become their more colourful counterparts, 'hype and horror'; why complex issues become reified into black and white; why complex issues become encapsulated in a sound bite which can then mask, rather than illuminate, the issues it aims to signify; 'designer babies', 'Frankenstein foods'. To an extent, the media also reports what it is told, for which it cannot necessarily be blamed: if 'experts' say there will be jam tomorrow, this will be reported in the media; depending on the specific article and the context, more or less attention will be paid to counter-claims or deconstructions of such statements. 'Gene for' stories are less common now in media reports, as the science itself develops and re-tells its own narrative.

Horlick-Jones, Walls, Katzinger *et al.* (2007) discuss how publics are not passive audiences but are extremely able to 'read' the media, bringing their life experience to the headline and the article; a capacity they term 'bricolage'. The ability of publics to apply life experiences in different contexts to their 'reading' of media headlines and news stories is cause for optimism. However, this is not to be complacent and to say that media-savvy publics can thus be safely left to navigate through media framings and arrive at balanced meanings. Media debates are framed in specific ways, which reflect the aims and remit of the medium. The framing of debates is central to which issues are discussed, how stakes are set, who is enrolled as a stakeholder and an 'expert', and whether mature discussions ensue. Ambivalence is often 'framed out' of media stories; and other ways of framing the discussion along broader lines, are often also missed.

Conclusion

This chapter has provided an account of the qualitative methodologies used to provide and analyse the data in this book, and explained the use of theoretical tools such as Social Movement Theory for understanding public engagement. The chapter further reiterated the difference between public engagement as social movement, and public engagement as policy practice. It has set out an overview of the publics engaging with human genetics which were traced during the timeframe 2003–6/7, with a particular focus on case study UK 'sustainability citizenship' networks and patient groups. These 'cast list' introductory overviews provide some snapshots of a highly complex, very varied, very broad, emergent social field. Important debates on what public engagement is, what it is for, and who 'the public' are, have also been introduced to facilitate an understanding of how, why and in what circumstances, different publics engage with human genetics. The following chapters tell contextualised stories of which publics are engaging with specific issues, how they engage with them and why, starting with UK public engagement with human embryonic stem cell research in chapter 2.

2 Stem cells and cloning

Introduction

This chapter provides a narrative account of human embryonic stem cell (hESC) research, giving examples of how a number of different publics have engaged with it during 2003–7 – what sorts of public debates have been had, how they have been 'framed' and by whom. It identifies what research has been carried out, how a regulatory framework has been constructed around the science, and what the hopes and expectations of the science are. The UK is at the forefront of encouraging such research and its legislature has facilitated this. Policy facilitation, scientific research and the particular significance accruing to the use of human embryos, means that hESC have been the focus of much of the public engagement in the UK in the timeframe covered by this book and it is thus hESC which is the primary focus of this chapter.

hESC research is seen by patients, many scientists and policy makers, as a potential therapy for some named diseases, a potential route for tissue and cell replacement, and as an important resource for further R&D. The chapter gives some examples of how different publics, including policy makers, have 'framed' the debate, identifying that some issues and frames are very loudly heard, such as the tendency for the debates on hESC to be reduced to 'cures or embryos'. Discourses of hope and opposition relating to the use of the human embryo are common; however other publics are framing a more complex and ambivalent set of risks and concerns relating to the use of women's bodies as a source of hESC.

This chapter is divided into two sections. The first section provides a narrative account of what stem cells are, and what research is being done on them, focusing on hESC. The second section focuses more on a specific case study; policy shifts by the Human Fertilisation and Embryology Authority (HFEA) in 2006–7 to allow 'egg sharing' and 'altruistic egg donation' for cloning to create hESC for research. This section first identifies the 'usual suspect' pro and anti framings of hopes for cures by patient groups, set against 'pro-life' concerns about the status of the embryo; discourses which have set the tone for public debate. The second part of this section provides a detailed account of responses from feminists to HFEA policy shifts in 2006–7, identifying that these prime movers provided a more complex and ambivalent set of issue frames relating to the use of women's bodies in biomedical research.

Section one: a stem cell narrative

What are stem cells and what are they 'for'?

Stem cell research is not per se a genetic technique, but it is closely associated with several genetic techniques. It is included as a key chapter in this book because the boundaries between different biomedical fields have become much less clear; this is the interconnected 'techno-science' described in the introduction. From 2003–7 in the UK, stem cell research was most often associated with the use of human embryos, from which a specific type of stem cells – human embryonic stem cells (hESC) – can be derived/extracted.

Stem cells from animals, and 'adult' stem cells from human and animal sources, are also the focus of much research, especially in countries which had, or do have, partial or complete bans on hESC research such as America,[1] Germany and Spain (Schneider 2007). Adult stem cells are found in major organs of the body, for example, in the liver and the skin, in bone marrow and birth cord blood. In November 2008 in Barcelona, the latest of a long line of vaunted stem cell 'breakthroughs' occurred; the reprogramming of adult skin cells to make stem cells was named by the journal *Science* (2008) as its 'breakthrough of the year'. It may well be the case that adult stem cells will leapfrog over hESC as the focus of research. The potential for the 2008 'Barcelona breakthrough' was already being discussed by savvy 'prime movers' in 2005, who framed hESC as being a research process means to an end, rather than a specific therapy end in itself:

> you'll produce the knowledge [through hESC research] and the knowledge will eventually be used to re-programme adult stem cells to re-differentiate them.
>
> ('Peter')

During 2003–7, many 'prime movers' were thus making an important distinction between hESC as a research process potentially leading to further research 'breakthroughs'; as opposed to hESC used as a potential therapy in and of itself.

Certain types of stem cells are 'pluripotent'; that is, they have the capacity to develop, or differentiate, into different types of cells; and this pluripotency is what has catalysed the expectation about what stem cells can deliver. Stem cells derived in whole or in part from a specific human donor have the potential to be used to treat that specific person if they had a particular disease or condition. This might overcome current problems of auto-immune rejection of organs and tissue experienced by patients, because the introduced tissue grown from this source would be a genetic 'match' for the donor.[2] Stem cells can not only differentiate, they can also be encouraged to replicate; the results of such replication are 'stem cell lines', which provide a source of stem cells which are 'banked' (see chapter 3) – that is, stored under regulated conditions,– and used as the basis of a number of R&D processes.

Box 2.1
Human Embryonic Stem Cells Timeline

1978 First baby (Louise Brown) born via IVF.

1984 Warnock report defines the 'primitive streak' enabling scientists to use embryos (termed blastocysts or 'pre-embryos') up to 14 days old.

1998 US scientist first differentiates hESC (Thomson *et al.* 1998).

1998 Dolly the sheep cloned at Roslin Institute.

2002 House of Lords debates stem cell research.

2003 hESC (derived from discarded embryos) reported as replicating in UK making 'stem cell lines'.

2004 HFEA grants first licence for cloned human embryos to be created specifically for hESC research.

2004/5 Hwang 'breakthrough' – claimed to have created hESC from cloned human embryos.

2006 Hwang research found to be fraudulent.

2007 HFEA policy makes it possible for women to trade eggs in return for IVF, or to donate eggs. Eggs are specifically for the creation of hESC.

2007 House of Lords debates stem cell research for second time.

2008 HFEA Act passed in Parliament has exceptionally broad terms, allowing a number of reproductive and cloning techniques.

Many scientific researchers and their supporters hope that stem cells could provide therapies for a range of diseases, including the following which are consistently named; Huntington's, Alzheimer's, Parkinson's, type 1 diabetes, cystic fibrosis and heart disease (*Time* 2009). Therapies are envisaged in the form of new nerve cells and tissue grown from stem cells introduced directly into the patient to replace and regenerate cells that the disease has destroyed. Stem cells could be a source of tissue to enable diseased organs to self-heal. Stem cells could also be used to test the effects of different drugs in relation to specific conditions (chapter 4), particularly the effects of drugs on stem cells derived from sources with a specific genetic trait, for example the 'single gene disorder' Cystic Fibrosis (Burnham 2009). This melding of genetic techniques with basic stem cell research shows how 'wet bench' basic research and applied techniques are merging together, blurring the lines between research and application and creating techno-scientific 'hybrid objects' (Latour 1993).

Despite the promissory nature of many scientific and media pronouncements, all stem cell research is in an early stage of development, where much is unknown, uncertain and yet to be consistently replicated, and there is little in the way of applied treatments beyond highly experimental one-offs in exceptional circumstances (UKSCF 2009) and reports of experimental, unregulated, hESC therapies in Russia (AP 2005) and India (*The Age* 2008). This comment from 'Ian' in 2004 is still current: 'We've got stem cell research going on, but ... there's not ... a direct therapeutic application at this stage.'

In a conference in 2007,[3] a representative from the UK stem cell bank noted that even the conditions under which stem cell lines were stored at the bank represented important variables which necessitated further research; for example, should the lines be stored in a fridge with a glass door allowing some light to fall on them, or in the dark? The uncertainty of the science and appliance of stem cells is an important aspect of their narrative. Health and environmental risks and uncertainties accruing to the use of stem cells have been identified by many 'prime movers'. In summary, people have asked how safe and reliable the science is, for example how would stem cells introduced into a patient's body actually behave? This is uncertain. There are examples of tumours developing in French children treated via gene therapy for their leukaemia (Bowring 2003). There is also some uncertainty about whether there might be potentially irreversible impacts on the genomes of patients who have had stem cells introduced into their bodies. There is a further potential medical/health risk to the patient in relation to auto-immune rejection responses to the stem cell material, and/or to the genetically modified virus 'transmitting' the material (Bowring 2003; Ho 2003). Others, such as the campaign group Institute for Science In Society (ISIS) have discussed the risk and uncertainty relating to unpredictable potential for environmental impacts and accruing population impacts. For example, the accidental release of viral vectors associated with the introduction of stem cells into the body could have severe consequences for the environment and population health (Ho 2003).

Human embryonic stem cells (hESC)

'Adult' stem cells can be derived from anyone, often in relatively straightforward procedures. However the creation or acquisition of hESC specifically is not straightforward in any sense. Eggs and embryos usually exist inside a woman's body; if they exist outside it, this means that a number of techniques have been enrolled to extract eggs and to make embryos, and this generates much controversy in relation to hESC research. Following the controversial identification of the 'primitive streak' in the Warnock report (1984),[4] embryos are allowed to develop for up to 14 days before development is halted. Embryos in this very early developmental stage are generally referred to as 'blastocysts' or 'pre-embryos', and it is when they are at this stage that further R&D takes place such as the derivation of stem cell lines from the embryo. Terminology is hugely important and highly contested, as Section two discusses in relation to egg 'sharing'; Mulkay (1993) provides an account of the easing of the legislative pathway through the development of the term pre-embryo; see also Spallone (1988).

hESC come from the following sources:

- from embryos created for IVF purposes, but not implanted (for a variety of reasons).
- from embryos created through Somatic Cell Nuclear Transfer; 'therapeutic cloning'.
- from the creation of 'hybrid embryos'.

In 2003, the first successful hESC lines (hESC cells which had been made to replicate) were derived from specific types of human embryos. These were embryos which had been genetically screened for specific conditions – the technique known as Preimplantation Genetic Diagnosis (PGD) (chapter 5) – and rejected for In Vitro Fertilization (IVF) purposes when found to carry the specific disease-carrying gene. In their paper announcing the successful creation of stem cell lines, Pickering *et al.* (2003) emphasised the significance of embryos discarded following PGD as providing a source of hESC. An immediate scientific/medical concern was the question of whether a stem cell line derived from PGD-rejected embryos carrying a specific genetic trait was itself going to express the genetic trait; in other words, would 'faulty' embryos create 'faulty' lines? This uncertainty was partially responsible for the ongoing search to derive hESC by other means.

A second means of creating hESC is so-called 'therapeutic cloning' to create a cloned embryo.[5] Using a technique sometimes known as Cell Nuclear Transfer (CNT) and sometimes Cell Nuclear Replacement (CNR), a human egg is stripped of its nucleus, and the nucleus replaced by a human cell, to create a cloned human embryo. A cloned embryo created by CNT could in theory be implanted into a human female body and carried to term; this is human reproductive cloning. This is currently banned in many countries, although certain 'mavericks' have courted global media controversy by claiming to have carried this out in countries with no such ban (BBC 2004a). Animal reproductive cloning is now regularly carried out, for example the creation of cloned mice and the infamous clone 'Dolly' the sheep (Einsiedel *et al.* 2003; Franklin 2007) which heralded the clone age. In the case of human therapeutic cloning for the derivation of hESC, the embryo created by CNT is then used for stem cell R&D. The HFEA first granted licences for this technique in 2004. In what has been referred to as 'Hwang-gate' (Franklin 2008), the work of the Korean scientist Woo Suk Hwang, who claimed to have successfully derived hESC stem cell lines via CNT and whose peer-reviewed research was published in *Science*, and *Nature*, to global acclaim, was subsequently found in 2006 to have been fraudulent (*Nature* 2006a). Despite this body blow, subsequent research on CNT-derived hESC lines has moved from being a speculative practice to becoming a more assured technique.

Aiming to provide a primarily factual narrative of what stem cell research *is*, this account has so far deliberately skimmed over the minefields associated with the derivation and use of hESC from any source, which have been the subject of much public debate. However the scientific narrative merges with political, social, ethical and legal narratives at certain points so completely that it is impossible not to at least flag issues which will be returned to later in the chapter. A key example of this is the fallout from 'Hwang-gate', where challenges to the ability of peer-reviewed 'sound science' to operate effectively as regulated, viable scientific practice catalysed the further development of specific regulatory frameworks and bodies, not least in the UK (Franklin 2008). Another important fallout from 'Hwang-gate' was the emergent public controversy over the source of the eggs used for his research. Some of the eggs had apparently been taken from junior female researchers amongst Hwang's own staff (HOOO 2006), and this consent process has been strongly criticised (Magnus and Cho 2006). Concerns about the acquisition of human eggs for hESC research generally became a 'line in the sand' moment for a number of feminists in 2005–7, discussed in Section two.

How human eggs are acquired for cloning to create hESC was, and remains, an exceptionally important ethical problem. It is also a logistical problem, as the scarcity of availability of human eggs combined with the experimental nature of the research means that

> there's not going to be the eggs to make all these [personalised treatments] ... if you're suffering from liver failure you would have to find an egg ... And where is that going to come from? ... there's already a shortage of eggs ... we really mustn't over hype the potential benefit [of hESC].
> ('Peter')

The scarcity of availability of human eggs has played a part in the third potential route for creating hESC; the creation of cloned 'hybrid' human/animal embryos, using CNT to create the cloned hybrid from a rabbit's or cow's egg and a human cell (*The Times* 2006). The scientist Stephen Minger has been pioneering this technique in the context of his research on degenerative disorders such as Parkinson's and type 1 diabetes (KCL 2004).

Minger's hybrid embryos as a potential source for hESC became one of the main media stories of 2008 (*The Times* 2008a).

To recap, then, discarded embryos, cloned human embryos created specifically for stem cell research, and cloned human/animal hybrid embryos, are currently the three key routes by which UK research is focused in relation to hESC. Despite the 'future promise', cloning routes for hESC creation are still highly experimental, and hESC from 'discarded' embryos is still currently the most reliable route for creating hESC stem cell lines.

Stem cell regulation and policy

In November 2008 the UK radically revised the HFEA Act and remit through a parliamentary Act (Dept of Health 2008c), in the process closing a number of regulatory gaps to provide very broad, blanket cover for a range of research procedures and techniques relating to reproduction and embryology (see also chapter 5) including stem cells, cloning, and the use and screening of human embryos. Current and future legislation, research directions and public responses, have arisen and will arise out of previous social engagement and the legacy of past research; the 2008 Act was thus the direct consequence of the state of play during the timeframe 2003–7, and of course the legacy of previous legislation and debate.

This broad remit has replaced a case-by-case, patchy process of updating (some say creatively interpreting) the previous HFEA Act in specific contexts to allow for specific techniques and procedures. This piecemeal approach, from the perspective of frustrated pro stem cell research lobby groups, was seen to be 'holding up' research, and conversely by a range of other campaign groups critical of stem cell research for various reasons, as travelling in a one-way direction down a 'slippery slope', where anything and everything is allowed in the name of medical research. Pro research lobby groups such as 'Sense about Science' criticise regulatory processes as placing unnecessary, 'unethical' blocks on the race for cures;[6] whilst 'watchdog' campaign groups such as Human Genetics Alert criticise regulatory policy as simply acting to facilitate scientific practice by providing a framework within which it can legitimately operate. The academic Sarah Franklin notes that

> the UK ... [has] one of the most extensive regulatory frameworks for governance of assisted reproduction and embryo research anywhere in the world ... this widely emulated system, while highly bureaucratic ... is also one of the most tolerant, progressive, and liberal towards embryo research and ... hESC derivation.
>
> (Franklin 2008: 128)

These important debates on what regulation is and should be for, and associated debates on how it is doing, have consistently surfaced in public discourse on stem cell research, and are returned to later in this chapter.

EU regulatory frameworks also strike a note of carefully constructed confusion. The European Group on Ethics in Science and New Technologies (EGE), a body of 'expert stakeholders', was set up to advise the EU on biomedical issues including hESC-related research.[7] At least in part on the basis of EGE reports, in its Tissues and Cells Directive (CEC 2004) the EU took up an interesting political position which made statements identifying specific ethical concerns around the creation and use of hESC, while simultaneously enabling individual member countries to adopt their own legal and ethical positions on hESC research.

UK governance in this arena comprises a number of very interesting hybrids or 'assemblages' whereby in close consultation with regulation and policy, scientific research councils and other medical and scientific research, 'key stakeholders' are forming quasi-governance bodies concerned with developing 'best practice' around the derivation, storage and use of stem cell lines, including ethical issues accruing to the construction of informed consent criteria relating to the acquisition of bio-material; namely, eggs. A key example is the UK stem cell bank. On the recommendations of the 2002 Report of the House of Lords Select Committee on Science and Technology, The Medical Research Council (MRC) and the Biotechnology and Biological Sciences Research Council set up the publicly funded UK stem cell bank (UKSCB 2004), which has identified and set standards accruing to the sourcing, creation, storage and use of stem cell lines as a public resource. Franklin describes the banks' remit as 'a public, non-commercial, facility, which will provide a major resource for the global biotechnology community, including the commercial sector' (Franklin 2008: 130).

This rather begs the question, how a public resource which also provides a commercial service can be said to be non-commercial. Such confusion over the melding between public and private is a characteristic of modern technoscience. The UK stem cell bank is thus an important example of how stem cell 'science' is a politically networked, and socially located, hybrid space.

Franklin (2008) provides a narrative of the establishment in 2003 in the UK of a network called the Human Embryonic Stem Cell Coordinators (HESCCO), composed primarily of centres involved with hESC research, and also Assisted Conception Units (ACUs), namely infertility treatment centres which would potentially be sources of eggs for hESC research. It may be slightly inaccurate to characterise HESCCO and the UK stem cell bank as poachers turned gamekeepers, but this metaphor does work to flag up the significant fact that those most involved with the process of the 'wet bench' research and thus the most direct beneficiaries of the acquisition of eggs (leaving aside the potential for hESC to provide treatments and cures which might benefit others), are also highly influential in setting the ethical frameworks and stakes.

Such governance hybrid objects are also developing on the international scene. Informed directly by 'prime movers' from relevant UK bodies such as the UK stem cell bank, the International Society for Stem Cell Research's remit is similarly to provide benchmarks and best practice guidelines to which nations and research teams must adhere if they wish to participate. Again this remit straddles ambivalent territory between theoretically laudable aims of filling identifiable governance gaps, and concerns that those with a direct vested interest in the successful outcomes of such processes should be so wholly involved in framing and setting the ethical stakes.

To reiterate, this is not a definitive account of relevant regulatory and governance structures but one which identifies some of the key players. Again, because stem cell research represents a complex techno-scientific space consisting of multiple linked scientific and medical practices, a number of different regulatory bodies and bodies setting ethical stakes and 'best practice' relating to these different, linked, fields are also enrolled in their governance. HESCCO represents an important move towards developing these related links (between fertility and hESC research, in this case) into new forms of regulatory frameworks.

In terms of civil society input into regulation, pro-research lobby groups have good access, as do scientists in their roles as 'expert stakeholders'. For example, the pro research lobby group Progress Educational Trust won UK government funds to conduct online public debate in 2005 on stem cells (PET 2005). Access osmosis and boundary blurring between roles and spheres tends to occur predominantly between 'pro-research', 'pro-science' civil society stakeholders and governance. Other civil society 'stakeholders' are of course also inputting into governance through consultation and lobby processes, such as the pro-life group Comment on Reproductive Ethics (CORE). Other stakeholders, such as feminist groups and academics, have been less involved in direct input into governance and have mobilised elsewhere, constructing the debates in their own terms (Plows 2008b).

Section two. Case study: the HFEA 'Donating eggs' consultation and public responses, 2006–7.

In the UK, in 2006 the HFEA broadened its policy remit to enable the sourcing of human eggs from women specifically for the purpose of CNT to create hESC. A temporary licence was granted by the HFEA in response to specific requests for this procedure from the North East England Stem Cell Institute (NESCI) where following the granting of the licence in July 2006, stem cell scientist Alison Murdoch became something of a lightning conductor in that a gathering storm of feminist concern over the acquisition of human eggs found a focal point and a catalyst moment.[8] The terms of this licence were extended, then made into permanent policy in February 2007. Eggs can now be acquired for hESC derivation, subject to application to the HFEA for a license, via the following routes:

- 'Egg sharing': women 'share' (trade) some of their eggs in return for free IVF cycles.
- 'Altruistic donation' – eggs are taken from women not undergoing IVF.[9]

Timeline

- May 2006: HFEA gives a temporary licence to NESCI allowing IVF 'egg sharing' to create and research hESC.
- July 2006: Public consultation initiated by HFEA: *Donating eggs for research: safeguarding donors* (HFEA 2006).
- 21 December 2006: terms of 'temporary' licence given to NESCI extended by HFEA: women not already undergoing IVF can now donate eggs for hESC research.
- 21 February 2007: HFEA's decision makes both routes policy (subject to application to the HFEA (2007)).

The following sections describe some of the key public discourses and engagement which were current when the HFEA decision was made and were, in some cases, catalysed by this decision.

hESC and discourses of hope

During 2003–7, the UK patient groups[10] discussed in chapter 1 were identifiably pro stem cell research and were proactively lobbying for it. In different public settings, they framed promissory ('future promise') accounts of what stem cell science might deliver; namely cures and treatments. Several lobby and interest groups were also particularly vocal in their support for stem cell research, including Sense About Science, Progress Educational Trust and the Institute of Ideas. Amongst a range of tactics aimed at having a regulatory impact including significant interaction with relevant regulatory bodies and consultation processes, they lobbied extremely directly for stem cell research. A typical example of this type of pro stem cell discourse is the Association of Medical Research Charities' *Statement on Human Embryo and Stem Cell Research:*

> AMRC supported ... research on human embryos which was enabled in the UK in January 2001 by the extension of the Human Fertilisation and Embryology Act 1990. Many patients suffering from serious diseases, and infertile patients, could potentially benefit from this carefully regulated research.
>
> (AMRC 2003)

In interview, 'Susan' discussed how she and other UK prime movers have been lobbying for hESC research, developing European connections with other patient groups and, importantly, industry: 'We also get involved in issues like stem cell research ... we've been involved in [European lobbying] ... we have done this quite a lot in the past.'

'Susan' provides what might be termed a 'standard narrative' of hope and promise relating to stem cells, invoking all the people that could benefit ... the people that have Parkinson's and Alzheimer's where ... the stem cell technology could make such a difference to their lives, and all the other people ... who are going to be diagnosed in the future.

In the process of telling her story about her she became involved with campaign work, 'Susan' provides an account of the cloning of a mouse to carry the Cystic Fibrosis gene, and associated gene therapy research. In this process she invokes those (animal rights activists) who oppose the use of animals in medical research:

> Lawrence McGinty from ITN said ... they've got the mice and they're going to be doing gene therapy, what do you think about it? And I was saying I think this is wonderful, it's giving a better quality of life, hopefully for everybody. and I never thought [that] people actually are against this, they don't want mice to be used, they would rather the child died.

Susan also spoke about public opposition to the use of hESC specifically: '[and] the people that don't want embryonic cells taken ... you're stopped because a few people in the minority are against it, is that right? I don't think it is.'

This narrative emphasises clearly that stem cell debates are often polarised between 'pro and anti' positions, and framed as such by people taking a specific position. Interestingly, people (like 'Susan', in this example) who are understandably framing 'future promise' accounts, often themselves invoke or construct the voice of 'anti' positions, as a rhetorical means of situating their own position; here, 'Susan' assumes that those voicing criticisms would 'rather the child died'.

First-hand patient accounts were reported in the media, in relation to specific conditions, and the stories of individuals. 'Patients' as a type more generally were also invoked in media summary accounts of what stem cell research might do and who the beneficiaries might be. Similar mixes of first-hand patient accounts, claims made on behalf of patients, and often the naming of specific conditions with an implied potential benefit for those with these and other conditions, were common in relevant public policy literature, and the literature of relevant medical and scientific websites, especially ones with a high public profile:

> Stem cell research offers enormous potential for major advances in clinical therapy. Stem cells could be used to replace missing or damaged cells in important diseases, such as Diabetes and Parkinson's, and in the treatment of traumatic injury including paralysis. The establishment of the UK Stem Cell Bank is an important step along the way to realising this potential.
>
> (UKSCB 2004)

Note the amount of uncertainty framed in this quote ('could be'), coexisting with a discourse of 'future promise'. 'Future talk' is the focus of chapter 8.

A number of highly newsworthy 'breakthrough' and 'controversy' stem cell stories have emerged as media headline-grabbers (Haran *et al.* 2007). The Times made significant reference to the promissory framing of 'breakthroughs' in an editorial on stem cells:

> The word 'breakthrough' is much abused in reporting of medical research ... There are some advances, however, that genuinely stand out for their potential to change the course of human inquiry. The creation of versatile human stem cells from reprogrammed adult tissue, which has just been named by the journal 'Science' as its Breakthrough of the Year, is certainly amongst them.
>
> (*The Times* 2008e)

'Breakthrough' discourse in media stem cell reportage can relate both to the technique itself, such as cloning, and to identified potential application of the research; generally treatments and cures for specific named diseases. Narrative accounts of 'breakthroughs' which may help patients are then 'balanced' by opposing views, with an overall aim of identifying risks and benefits. In the case of stem cells, oppositional voices are readily on hand, loudly opposing hESC research; namely, 'pro-life' groups. Easy-to-follow narratives of 'cures or embryos' thus dominate media accounts of hESC research, much to the frustration of campaign groups wishing to make more complex points which do not fit neatly into this 'for or against' narrative and which are often 'framed out' of most media accounts, in a constantly reiterative process.

hESC and discourses of opposition

Anti abortion (popularly termed 'pro life') campaigners have been extremely vocal in their opposition to any research which uses human embryos, including the use of 'discarded' PGD embryos, and human cloning to create hESC. A very important 'prime mover' group is Comment On Reproductive Ethics (CORE).

> CORE is a public interest group focusing on ethical dilemmas surrounding human reproduction, particularly the new technologies of assisted conception ... Absolute respect for the human embryo is a principal tenet ... the group has been involved in ... lobbying against human cloning.
>
> (CORE ca. 2005)

A mixture of pro-life and religious opposition to hESC in relation to the ethics of research on the human embryo, is a social account which has dominated the public debates, not least the framing of the issues at stake in the regulatory sphere. In the 2002 and 2007 House of Lords debates (Hansard

2002, 2007a) on stem cell research and again in the 2008 parliamentary debates leading to the revision of the HFEA Act (Hansard 2008), and in accompanying media reportage, the ethics of the use and status of human embryos dominated accounts of what issues were at stake. Not all 'pro-life' campaigners are religious, and similarly not all religious groups are 'pro-life', and there is a danger of reducing what is actually quite a complex set of actors into a reified position which does not represent social reality. A religious or ethically informed concern about use of the human embryo, does not mean that one is by default 'pro-life and anti-abortion, although this is definitely the position of the Catholic church, for example. In contrast, religious perspectives expressed in the UK in relation to stem cell research, often tend to be pro reproductive choice, and essentially humanist in outlook; not stridently 'against' hESC, still less 'anti science', but rather identifying how hESC research catalyses important philosophical questions on human nature and human identity, as 'James' identifies:

> what is the embryo? Is it just the broad cells, or is it as human as a baby is, or is it something in between? ... what the Catholic, Orthodox and some Christians are saying is that [an embryo] gets the same rights as a baby; i.e. don't do any research ... The other extreme is that [the embryo] has no functional meaning. It's a 'brick', somebody once described it ... Very few critics would take that view of things.
>
> ('James')

Discussions of the moral status of the embryo are complex and draw upon a heady mix of scientific findings and moral and theological arguments, including views about the status of women, together with pragmatic considerations. The Catholic church, as well as others, dates the formation of a unique human being at the point of conception: the point at which all the genetic material which will go on to form an independent individual comes together. This has not always been the case; when less was known about the scientific aspects of pregnancy and embryonic development, the church took a much looser view of the status of the embryo and fetus. In any case, from a religious point of view, what is important is the point of ensoulment, the point at which a unique human soul becomes embodied. Killing an embryo at any point therefore is the killing of a human individual and hence prohibited in official church doctrine. In practice, many identifying themselves as Catholics depart from this view. Other major religions take alternative views, for instance, the Muslims consider that ensoulment takes place at 120 days after conception (Daar and Khitamy 2001).

The synod of the Church of England, when discussing these issues, considered the formation of a nurturing relationship between embryo and mother crucial and picked on the point of implantation as the start of life.

The Warnock report in 1985 fixed upon the formation of the 'primitive streak', the precursor of the nervous system, as the cut-off point for allowing an embryo to develop *in vitro*. This compromise can be seen to have stemmed from a secular view of the worth of a human being focused upon our mental attributes, together with pragmatic considerations about research needs.

The status of the human embryo is an important and emotive issue, and it is not only Catholics, other religions, and pro-life-ers, who express varying shades of concern, distaste and opposition to the use of human embryos; but of course these voices are extremely prevalent in the debates. Research on the human embryo is a 'boundary object' (Star and Griesemer 1989) which touches many people, as it is tied up with issues of human-ness and human identity, what it means to be human, whether there is anything 'special' about the creation of a human life. Many secular humanists, not to mention many of the 'general public', demonstrate a spectrum of concerns ranging from support, abhorrence, to indifference, to secular philosophical musings. Despite the very loud, polarised, clash of 'cures vs embryos', people have the capacity to demonstrate ambivalence, to feel multiple things at once. To be uncomfortable about the use of human or hybrid embryos in research does *not* make one 'pro-life' by default, and many people voice concerns or objections while also being sympathetic to the needs of patients for cures. Similarly, findings on public views on hESC research carried out by the MRC in 2002 noted that

> Generally the non-IVF [focus group] participants accepted the use of embryos at a very early stage of development. However, people who had received IVF treatment had quite different views of embryos; the women in particular, viewed embryos as babies and their frozen embryos as potential siblings for their existing children. The creation of embryos for research was generally rejected, whether this was by IVF procedures using eggs and sperm or by cell nuclear transfer (CNT).
>
> (PSP 2004)

This ambivalence, a key theme throughout the book, is not easily heard when debates are framed in terms of 'pro or anti', as interviewees tended to point out: 'the [stem cell] debate has been framed in a certain way, you're either for or against ... so other issues, other considerations ... cannot be expressed' ('Lucy').

The 'stem cell debate' often gets reified into what Mulkay (1993) termed 'rhetorics of hope and fear in the great embryo debate'. This for or against framing of the stakes is perpetuated

- by the regulatory system
- by the media
- by prime movers in the debates themselves (such as patients and 'pro-lifers')

'Lucy' noted how a specific type of regulatory structure framed the debate:

our legal system is for or against, our parliamentary system has been a binary for and against ... whereas in Holland for instance the political decision making [process] is much more consensus [based].

('Lucy')

The debate is framed by patient prime movers as a choice between hope/cures/treatments, and people who have concerns about the use of animals or human embryos. Such patient groups are at loggerheads with those who have ethically entrenched positions relating to the use of human embryos, or the use of animals. However this clash of 'lifeworlds' has the result of turning some extremely complex debates into 'usual suspect' black and white ones. Especially with such emotive issues at stake – such as the possibility of stopping the premature death of a young person with CF, for example – it becomes incredibly difficult to voice an ambivalent position: 'if you raise questions, [it looks as if] you want people to suffer and die'('Lucy').

'Pro-life' opposition to hESC research has been a loudly heard frame, in part because the simplicity of the claim makes for a simple narrative easily grasped in a complex space: this translates, in general terms, as 'pro cures or pro life?', or, 'patients or embryos'. This highly polarising framing of individuals' position in the stem cell debate as being one of support or opposition to hESC on the basis of the status of the human embryo (important though this issue is, for many people, not just pro-life groups), has also 'framed out' the perspectives of other groups with critical positions, who do not fall neatly into this either/or account of stem cell research. As a result, there is a default discourse which rolls into play when the issue comes up in the public sphere; namely that to voice concerns, one is anti cures. In this environment, a possible reason why other (UK) publics are not coming forward to voice concerns is because of this polarised and reified framing of the debate. This is counter-productive to having mature debates about the science and the associated multiple overlapping issues such as risk, medical viability, the role of governance. There is room for ambivalence; one can be, for example, supportive of patients' hopes for treatments, and still voice concerns and caveats. Such debates are important for 'cross talk' between perspectives.

In this chapter the volume has been turned down, so to speak, on the pro-life narrative and the 'status of the embryo versus patients' needs' framing of the debates, in order to highlight other issues, perspectives and voices which seek to re-frame the debate on stem cells along different track lines, and/or who identify shades of grey in this often polarised debate. It is to these lesser heard discourses that we now turn.

'Tilting the frame': complex (feminist) responses to the 2006 HFEA consultation

A legacy of feminist activism in the Women's Health Movement and academic feminist critiques of the representation/exploitation of women's bodies in relation to the use of the female body in science and medicine (Spallone 1992; Haraway 1991) is being re-addressed by a number of contemporary academics, specifically in the context of stem cell research (Throsby 2004; Franklin and Roberts 2006; Nahman 2006, Sexton 2001, 2005; Dickenson 2002, 2007; Schneider 2007; Parry 2006; Haran and O'Riordan 2006; O'Riordan and Haran 2009). There is a particular type of feminism being articulated here, which might be termed 'eco-feminist' (Mies and Shiva 1993) in its linking of social and environmental justice ('sustainability citizenship') issues, with those of women's rights, women's bodies and associated risks. Women are in the front line, having to negotiate new territory; they are 'moral pioneers' (Rapp 1999). These feminists are raising concerns relating to why, how, where, under what conditions, human eggs are being derived for research, framing the questions in terms of issues of gendered risk; the trade (and hence power) relationships between the producers and consumers of bio-products, namely eggs, with significant 'bio-value' (Waldby 2002). They also frame broader questions about routes to population health, and issues around citizenship and public engagement.

ReproKult, for example, is a highly mobilised campaign group based in Germany, drawing together academics, medical professionals such as mid-wives, and other feminist campaigners, who during 2003–7 were proactively building international network links.

> ReproKult wants to raise awareness of the social implications of new medical technologies, especially for women, and criticizes narrow, embryo-centric discourses.
>
> (ReproKult 2005)

During 2005–6, 'prime movers' from these specific campaign groups and broader networks developed an increasingly vocal critique of the use of women's eggs. Information was circulated via campaign nodes such as ReproKult, and triggered increasing controversy not only among more under-ground networks of eco-feminist anti capitalist activists, but also amongst academic networks. In the UK and indeed across Europe, these informal networks were catalysed into action when in July 2006, the HFEA released the *Donating Eggs* public consultation document. The HFEA policy moves catalysed criticism related specifically to the extraction and use of women's eggs for hESC research. This was a discourse relating primarily to the use of the female body and the construction of gendered risk. It also raised questions about policy practice. These issues were set out in a jointly signed open letter, written by some feminists and other 'prime movers', to the *Guardian* in May 2006.

> We are very concerned about the proposal to allow cloning researchers to collect eggs from women who are not undergoing IVF ... and who will receive no therapeutic benefit. We are in favour of women's rights to

control their bodies and their fertility. We believe that the risks of hor-
monal hyperstimulation of the ovaries cannot be justified in basic
research, in which the benefits are very uncertain: the risk/benefit ratio is
far too high ... We call on the HFEA to reject this proposal, which
represents a significant danger to women's health, and is a form of
exploitation of women's bodies.

(*Guardian* 2006)

This letter signalled a broader movement by certain UK feminist academics
and others to critically articulate concerns and opposition relating to this
issue in the public sphere. Several events took place in 2006 bringing together
concerned feminist academics and civil society stakeholders to discuss egg
collection and the HFEA consultation (Plows *et al.* 2006). The following sub-
sections provide more detail about the key concerns and issues raised by these
groups, networks and individuals in direct response to the terms of the HFEA
consultation.

In its consultation, the HFEA used the terms 'egg sharing' and 'donation'
to describe the transaction of a woman providing eggs either in return for
IVF or 'altruistically donating'. Terms are important and these have been
strongly critiqued. The feminist bioethicist Donna Dickenson has described
the IVF transaction as a 'trade'. Because of the increasing use of IVF in
the UK and globally (Bharadwaj 2005), increasing numbers of women are
likely to encounter the IVF egg trade arrangement. Also, some women in
countries outside the UK are simply selling their eggs for UK hESC research.
Sexton (2005) charts the route of eggs from Romania (see also Nahman
2006), and highlights concerns about exploitation of economically marginalised
women.

Eggs are an important 'bio-resource' with 'bio-value'. The prioritising of
'bio-competitiveness' and the marketing of bioscience for economic growth
has been described as the 'bio-economy' (Birch 2006) (chapter 4). Addressing
the Royal Society in 2006, Tony Blair said:

If we do not take the opportunities that are there for us in science, then
we are not going to have a successful modern economy ... [I]t is at the
cutting edge of science that our human capital can be most exploited for
our country's future.

(Blair 2006)

In response, 'sustainability citizenship' prime movers have criticised the remit
of 'the bio-economy', for example, in relation to the social and ethical
impacts of global trade in human resources. The language of exploitation is
significant. Several commentators have critiqued the commodification of the
female body (Sexton 2005; Dickenson 2002, 2007; Schneider 2007), where
women's bodies are the site for the exploitation of resources with identified
'bio-value'.

An ongoing debate within feminism is whether women can really give 'informed consent' in this specific context, or conversely whether is it patronising to question their ability to do so. Informed consent criteria relating to women who might 'share' or 'donate' [trade] eggs for hESC research formed an important part of the 2006 HFEA consultation. However critics argued that the terms of the consultation failed to locate the broader political and social background against which 'informed consent' in a specific context is given by a specific woman. For example, the proposed informed consent criteria for a woman motivated to trade her eggs for 'free' IVF cycles does not take into account the background factor of the cultural stigma of infertility which may be influencing a woman's decision to consent to this arrangement. The uncertainty over long-term health outcomes also has implications for the viability of patients giving 'informed consent' to these procedures.

'Choice' is another important, highly characteristic, aspect of the way debates on egg collection for hESC research were framed in the HFEA consultation. The framing of the procedure in terms of (reproductive) choice has been heavily contested, as it situates those who critique the procedure as 'anti choice'. In the *Guardian* letter given above, the authors made it clear that opposition to egg donation did not make them 'anti-reproductive choice'. Choice and consent in relation to the HFEA consultation are further discussed in chapter 7.

A discourse of gendered altruism (egg donation) is also embedded within the HFEA policy document. Using similar discourses to blood and organ donation, concepts of 'duty' and 'citizenship' (discussed further in chapters 3 and 6) and appeals to the 'public good' are being invoked in relation to genetics, reproduction and fertility, from key regulatory and scientific sources (Plows and Boddington 2006). Despite the uncertainty accruing to stem cell research, a 'default setting' position is that science and scientific knowledge will provide answers and solutions, and thus 'supporting science' amounts to a public duty.

There are however major differences in terms of the potential risks accruing to such altruism, between different types of public donation of bio-material. In the context of egg 'donation', a very obvious point is simply that women specifically are taking this risk; it is 'gendered'. In order to harvest multiple eggs from women, drugs are given to stimulate the ovaries so that several eggs are released at once. A reaction to the drugs, known as ovarian hyperstimulation, affects one in ten women undergoing this procedure; the condition can be fatal in rare cases. Health uncertainty is also an issue, as the long-term impacts of drugs are unknown (*Nature* 2006b).

As the timeline at the start of Section two shows, the initial 'temporary' licence granted by the HFEA pre-dated the launch of the public consultation. Further, on 21 December 2006 the HFEA extended this temporary licence to NESCI while the public consultation process on the topic was ongoing. This is a case of regulation putting the cart before the horse (Plows 2007b). In

several settings, critical points relating to the viability of this public consultation process have been raised, which can be summarised as:

- How well the public was informed; the public consultation consisted of a
  confusing, highly complex document; this was not a proactive effort to
  meaningfully engage 'the general public' and falls short of identified best
  practice.
- Whether the HFEA's response to the consultation was a *fait accompli*.
- How the consultation 'framed' the debate.

In relation to this last bullet point, the consultation document asks the basic
question: should 'altruistic donation' be allowed? But the subtitle of the
document, 'Safeguarding donors' shifts the terms of the consultation to
assume that it should be allowed, moving the focus of consultation to protecting donors from harm. Questions inside the document relate to donor risk
management, for example through 'informed consent' procedures.

The pre-emptive nature of the temporary licence extension by the HFEA in
December 2006, and the framing of the document, catalysed and re-framed a
crisis in confidence in (UK) public engagement and consultation mechanisms.
These are 'classic' Science and Technology Studies (STS) and public understanding of science (PUS) issues (Wynne 1996, 2006; Jasanoff 1990) which
can be summarised as being a contestation of the legitimacy of policy practice
by different publics/citizens. In other words, what is regulation *for*? 'Regulation works because it gives credence' ('Lucy'). What gets discussed and passed
as law or policy helps set up the terms of what specific issues and technological manifestations people encounter and how they debate it. This is triggering a recurring question, especially amongst activists critical of the way
human genetics as a set of technologies is being produced, namely: 'is regulation therefore just a fig leaf on the free market model, whereby markets
dictate techno-scientific moves and governance struggles to keep up?' ('Lucy').
Franklin states that:

> Embryo research in the UK is ... protected by a stable regulatory envir-
> onment and a strongly positive government policy of support, which in
> turn are directly linked to promoting UK leadership in the 'knowledge
> economy' of the biosciences.
>
> (Franklin 2008: 128)

It is thus *not* a 'conspiracy theory' to state that the regulation aims to serve
the interests of the science in the further interests of the economy: this is its
stated agenda.

In 2003 it emerged that the 'pro-life' group CORE had been working with
certain feminists in the USA over stem cell research, identifying where their
respective critiques of the use of human eggs for research converged, while
continuing to differ over attitudes to abortion. This was an early sign of

emergent social complexity which developed during 2005/6 into an international campaign group, Hands Off Our Ovaries! (HOOO). HOOO is a significant 'hybrid object' emerging from the techno-social space of stem cell research; an important signifier of social ambivalence in exceptionally complex terrain. HOOO's key frames relate to issues of political economy and gendered risk accruing to the acquisition of eggs, and do not in any clearly identifiable way mobilise the 'pro-life' opposition to hESC in terms of the human embryo, although the fact that CORE is involved with HOOO makes the 'pro-life' connection by default. Overall, feminist responses to HOOO have been mixed, at best, and in many cases downright critical, especially amongst younger feminist activists from countries such as Italy who continue to struggle against Catholic attitudes to abortion. Some UK feminists have asked why it was necessary to align with anti abortion campaigners, when the eggs issue had managed to achieve some visibility and space for matters pertaining to hESC which had nothing at all to do with the status of the embryo.

During the 'Emerging Politics' project a significant social phenomenon was identified which was termed 'strange bedfellows' (Evans *et al.* 2006), who can be summarised as a counter-intuitive cluster of social actors from different perspectives, different 'lifeworlds', who in highly context-dependent circumstances, may share, or appear to share, a position over a specific issue. These strange bedfellow hybrid publics are the result of a number of different factors. First they represent emergence: an early stage in the debates, where 'prime movers' and 'early risers' are still identifying the stakes. This is highly complex terrain where multiple issues interrelate, enabling or catalysing unusual convergences between normally oppositional 'lifeworld' positions. This is catalysing hybridity, as is an accompanying ambivalence 'beyond pro and anti'; that it is possible to hold multiple, conflicting positions, which provides the ground for convergences between perspectives. Last, there can be political pragmatism in terms of forming strategic alliances; for example, German feminists have a history of aligning with pro-life groups for political/legal rulings in the German parliament over reproduction (Schneider 2007).

The HOOO 'strange bedfellow' hybrid signals a significant phenomenon in public engagement with bioscience; that where stakes are multiple and complex, people from very different positions align and converge. Such hybrids are likely to be increasingly common, triggered through complexity and attempts at political pragmatism (at least as perceived by the participants) in terms of allowing an anticipated political result over a specific issue to take precedence over broader 'lifeworld' positions. The phenomenon of 'strange bedfellows' being catalysed in specific circumstances could be quite a commonplace social reality, and developing this potential perhaps enables more scope for explorations of nuance and complexity than the sociology of the clash of 'usual suspects' does. 'Strange bedfellows' are an interesting form of the types of hybrid convergences, the 'assemblages' (Irwin and Michael 2003) characterised by the blurring of boundaries between spheres, networks and individuals discussed in chapter 1.

Conclusion

This chapter has provided an overview of stem cell science, focusing on hESC, and giving a general outline of policy moves and accompanying public engagement. It has discussed the setting up of stem cell banks, a form of biobank (the subject of the next chapter) and identified forms of 'hybrid governance', which are also relevant to other typologies of biobanks, discussed further in chapter 3. It has identified that many issues being framed by 'prime movers' are failing to be heard clearly in the public arena (such as in media reportage of policy debates), most likely because they are complex and ambivalent frames, which don't work well in a space where publics are often put into polarised pro or anti positions; and where media and policy can frame the debate along narrow, pre-set lines. It is also hard to discuss ambivalence, when hopes and promises of cures and treatments for serious diseases are in the frame. The chapter has shown how some, such as certain feminists, have struggled to re-frame the stakes, for example to break out of the 'cures or embryos' paradigm, and raise issues of gendered risk accruing to the acquisition of eggs for hESC. The importance of how (and where, and on what terms, and by whom) the debate is framed, is flagged in the title of Sexton's (1999) paper, 'If cloning is the answer, what was the question?'

So, what is the question that cloning – and hESC research – is seen as the answer to, and who is asking that question? What hopes are attached to hESC? Is it how to exploit 'cutting edge' science for the benefit of 'UK plc', is it how to treat a specific disease, is it simply a wish to understand more about what stem cells can do? Or is the question more broadly, how can we be healthy as a society? Health is enrolled by prime movers who are pro stem cell research, as a promissory discourse where health is constructed in terms of disease, and stem cells are a potential cure for disease, often specified. Chapter 8 develops the issue of how the 'future promise' of bioscience is setting the policy agenda, and chapter 6 shows how many are framing this 'future promise' in terms of disease and condition cure and treatment, while others are questioning whether this is the best way to construct health and set health policy more generally. This is not about being 'anti stem cell research' but about interrogating how, and why, health priorities, strategies and provision (public budget-setting) are being established; and who is setting them, and what the fallout might be. There is an emergent debate on whether the melding of economic aims and agendas with health agendas is the best way to achieve health goals.

How, then, to debate ambivalence and complexity and move beyond either/or framings? More careful attention paid by those with the power to frame public debates would lead to more mature debates, which enabled discussion of relevant issues without people being forced into 'pro or anti science', 'pro or anti cures' artificial corners. However some would say if the whole point of regulation is to facilitate the science, why bother to take part in public consultation processes? Several interviewees had very cynical views of public consultation, saying that it is not in the interests of a governance framework explicitly set up to exploit bio-capital to give political space to those groups who are questioning this agenda. This is a theme which threads throughout the book in relation to the question of what 'public engagement' is and what it is for.

3   Biobanks and databases

Introduction

This chapter focuses on two high profile, large biobanks/databases in the UK: the UK Biobank, instigated by the Wellcome Trust, which has a primary 'medical' (health) focus; and the police national DNA database (NDNAD) which has a primary 'non-medical' goal of tackling crime. Much of the emergent UK regulatory framework governing biobanks and databases has been catalysed because of these two key collections. Biobanks have also been the focus of a significant amount of public engagement, mostly from patient groups, and genetic and civil liberties watchdogs. The chapter is divided into two sections. Section One provides an overview of the typologies and remits (aims and objectives) of different types of biobanks and databases. Section Two focuses specifically on the Wellcome biobank and the NDNAD.

In providing these narratives, the chapter gives an overview of some of the many publics who are engaging with the issue of biobanks and databases in the public sphere, identifying the key ways in which they frame, or set the stakes of, the debate. Because biobanks are a means to an end, publics identified in this cast list are often commenting on the actual and potential *end use(s)* or goal(s), and associated risks and benefits, of the biobanks and databases – for example disease cures, treatments and prevention; stigma and discrimination, ownership and rights – as much they comment on the terms (means) of the biobank/database itself. These are of course connected as means dictate ends; for example, whether a database is commercially owned; or the terms of informed consent given for use of sample data.

A number of organised public debates have taken place relating to the UK Biobank and NDNAD; run by Wellcome itself, by the UK Biobank Ethics and Governance Council, and also by civil society groups such as Progress Educational Trust. Besides the lobby groups and academics who turn up to these public events, however, the actual engagement by genuine 'members of the public' remains relatively small. There is also 'self-starting' public engagement in the form of various types of cultural, and bio-consumer, behaviour, catalysed by the broad range of biobanks and databases and the uses to which these are being put. A large amount of grassroots public engagement has been catalysed by the NDNAD, including the engagement of a number of race, children and civil liberties charities, organisations and individuals who have mobilised to express opposition and concern. The UK Biobank is also catalysing engagement by the 'general public' as potential sample donors.

Section one: a biobank narrative

A biobank is a collection of samples of biological material. Human biobanks consist of, for example, samples of blood, tissue or DNA extracted from these samples or skin swabs. There are also many animal and plant biobanks (APDB 2007). This chapter focuses on human biobanks, although the potential creation of biobanks of stem cell lines derived from hybrid human/animal embryos is blurring the distinction between animal and human in significant ways (chapter 2). The biobank can be broad/general; for example, a population-wide sample collection; or highly specific; for example, a database of samples from women who carry a specific breast cancer gene. A biobank consists of the biological sample itself. A database consisting of the digital information taken from the sample can operate/exist independently of the biobank of biological material from which the database is drawn; digital and biological banks and databases also operate/exist together. Because digitised DNA databases are derived from biobanks of samples, they are discussed in this chapter as on a continuum with biobanks. Databases of digitised information are increasingly the raw material for genetics research and development (R&D), through bio informatics searches, for instance (chapter 4).

Typologies of biobanks

According to leading research,

> The growth in genetic research has led to the establishment of a variety of genetic databases with different purposes … and sample collections established for single research projects. Despite this … there are no accepted definitions of 'genetic databases'.
> (Ethox 2005 website) For further information about the Ethox project, see Gibbons *et al.* (2007).

Difficulties with defining genetic databases and biobanks result from:

- Differences of size/scale. Banks vary from local micro samples to national/population biobanks (such as the UK Biobank), and international biobanks.
- Differences in typologies: biobanks and databases; biological and digital.
- Differences and confusion in articulated uses/remit: preventative, diagnostic, predictive, therapeutic, open-ended. The Wellcome Trust states that its biobank is for 'research purposes'.

- Differences in terms of ownership criteria, which range from private commercial to public non-profit, to public/private, to private non-profit.

In the UK, there is no definitive or standardised nomenclature, and little public debate about its absence. The UK Biobank, however, has been developing public consultation frameworks and running public engagement events in relation to its remit (Wellcome 2004, OECD 2006). Different types and sizes of biobanks generally imply different primary uses. The lack of clarity over typologies and proposed and potential uses of different biobanks/databases, has implications for regulation.

Box 3.1

Biobank and database key examples

All biobanks can potentially have associated digitised genetic databases, logging genetic information derived from the bio-material.

UK biobanks/databases examples

The list here is a mixture of general types, e.g. a biobank of blood samples, and specific examples, e.g. Virgin cord blood bank.

* blood samples - (for example, of Familial Hypocholestemia (FH))

* cancer tissue samples for specific research units

* Virgin cord blood bank[1] (a commercial biobank)

* egg freezing banks (can also be commercial)

* UK stem cell bank (chapter 2)

* sperm bank

* university/hospital databases

* UK population databases (Viking ancestry)

* UK 'disease community' biobanks and databases at micro and macro levels

* UK police DNA database (NDNAD)

* UK Biobank

International private biobanks/databases examples

* Iceland (privately owned, licensed by the Icelandic government – deCODE genetics, Inc.)[2]

* National Geographic and IBM private database of human genomic variation, The Genographic Project[3]

* Celera Corporation,[4] founded by Craig Venter – privately owned databases

International collaborative bio-database examples

* Human Genome Project

* ISSCR (international stem cell bank)

* HapMap (compiling a protein database – Single Nucleotide Polymers SNPs)

The range of typologies and remits is catalysing a great deal of engagement amongst different 'publics'. Some examples include:

• Sperm banks: as children born of sperm donation come of age, there is more discussion on their identity 'rights', particularly in relation to their genetic 'legacy'; UK legislation has recently been changed so that sperm donors are no longer guaranteed anonymity (Hansard 2004).
• Ancestry: 'who am I? where do I come from?' Public engagement has been triggered by projects such as the Genographic Project. Ancestry-focused genetic databases have also been given much publicity through UK 'reality TV' shows.
• Cancer biobank samples from specific cancers with a high genetic causality such as BRCA1 breast cancer; familial heritability patterns are triggering important forms of engagement within affected family relationships (chapter 5).
• Publics as 'bio-consumers': for example, parents wishing to store their baby's cord blood in the Virgin private bank in case this tissue later helps if any treatments are needed. The commercial sale of genetic tests to publics is discussed in chapter 5.

These are just some examples of the ways in which different types of bio-banks and databases are catalysing the engagement of specific types of publics, bio-consumers and patient groups. This is also triggering public debates (and assumptions) on identity, belonging to different types of (genetic) communities. These issues are discussed further in chapters 4, 5 and 6.

Overview of biobanks and databases research and development (R&D)

Why are samples stored and why is research carried out on them? Generally, medically (health) orientated research on sample data aims to understand disease expression, knowledge which could potentially be applied in predictive, diagnostic and therapeutic ways. This includes research on the samples of bio-material (blood, tissue), testing drugs, manipulating the sample, experimenting with environmental conditions, comparing/contrasting typologies within samples, and so forth. Stem cell line creation, storage and use discussed in chapter 2 is an example. Bio-infomatics (chapter 4) is a means of digitised genetic and genomic sequencing, enabling a search for genetic 'markers', repeats, patterns within samples. Sequenced samples can be used for specific and also general (open) searches. R&D is aiming to understand more about the extents and ways genetic, genomic (and proteomic) variables may contribute to disease/condition expression.

> say you've got a sequence and you don't know what the function [of that sequence] is ... If you can find some of its relatives in a gene, and more in another place in the human genome ... it will probably give you some clues as to the function of the gene.
>
> ('Alice')

Sequenced database samples could also be used for predictive mathematical modelling of known and/or uncertain variables. The developments in genetic, genomic and proteomic sequencing, and the associated R&D on biobanks and databases is linked to research on the Human Genome Project.[5,6]

The end uses of specific biobanks and databases vary considerably, depending on the type of sample, the aim of the specific biobank/database and its remit, the type of consent given and the way the biobank/database is set up and run. Examples include open public access, or private company, or small hospital lab, anonymised samples for broad research goals, or samples specifically taken to feed back to patients, and so on. Commercial service bio-banks (such as the Virgin bank which offers to store a baby's cord blood against possible future need) have a very different remit to that of a small or large-scale biobank of samples for medical research into a specific condition. For example 'single gene' disorders such as a specific form of breast cancer, or Cystic Fibrosis (CF), could have a biobank/database of samples which aim to target specifically that type of cancer. There are significant uncertainties and blurred boundaries in terms of future usage: from specific targeted aims, to open-ended 'secondary use' of samples and data. These projected uses can be (solely, simultaneously) diagnostic, predictive, therapeutic, curative.

Biobanks and databases as collections of samples are thus the means to various ends. The dominant articulated outcome for medical databases is disease identification, management, prevention, cure. A genetic test based on database/biobank research can identify disease/condition expression, on a spectrum from diagnostic in relation to the definite (identifying 'single gene' disorders) to predicting the possible ('susceptibility', 'predisposition'), and extremely tenuous. The predictive use of bio-information generated by bio-banks is a particular focus for critique by some 'prime movers'. Chapter 5 discusses genetic/genomic testing and screening in more detail. The development of targeted drugs relating to gene expression, and so-called 'personalised pharmaco', is discussed in chapter 4. Biobank and database information can be linked with other information, aiming to identify patterns in gene/environment interactions for example; this is known as genetic epidemiology.

Non-medical uses of biobanks/databases can be summarised as including:

- Policing – forensic and 'predictive' crime solving.
- Social/economic – workplace, insurance, paternity, ancestry.
- Bio-surveillance.
- Commercial activity (including development of medical products and patenting).

While there are major differences between 'non-medical' uses of biobanks and bio-databases and 'medical' ones, it is important to emphasise that these distinctions often blur in practice. Information taken for one purpose, for instance, could be used for another, such as police use of a medical database. Risks of stigma, discrimination and privacy breaches accruing to the use of someone's biological and genetic information are common to both medical and non-medical databases. The distinction between the two types of information is exceptionally blurred not only in terms of secondary use of data (GeneWatch 2006b; Cutter 2006), but also concerning 'medical and non-medical' uses. For example, health insurance, health targets, health budgets, medical and social policy strategies, based on 'susceptibility and predisposition', are all affected by the extent to which the information generated by biobanks and databases is relied upon (Dept of Health 2003). Differences between public and private ownership and use of samples is also a 'non-medical' issue which impacts on medical and health outcomes (for example, issues of access and benefit-sharing).

Many different products with commercial value can be derived from different types of biobanks and databases. Biobanks and databases are thus attracting much commercial interest, catalysing the emergent phenomenon of specific publics as bio-consumers; markets for the goods and services such biobanks can provide (chapters 4, 5); the capacity to store one's own bio-material, for example. The venture capitalist Richard Branson set up the Virgin newborn cord blood bank, providing a commercial public service. Google has invested in the genome mapping company '23 and me', potentially moving towards an online database (chapter 5). 'Big pharma' and associated research labs and spinout companies own many datasets and biobanks. Craig Venter's company Celera, for example, owns a number of bio and databases including genomic and proteomic samples. Chapter 5 discusses the commercial sale and use of genetic tests and genomic 'mapping' services in more detail.

The overall scientific accuracy and reliability of biobanks and databases is highly contested territory, because of this huge range of typologies and potential applications. Not only is there a variety of end uses and goals, ranging from diagnostic to predictive; there is also a tremendous range in how much of a role specific genes, or sets of genes, actually play in disease expression. Using biobanks for predictive purposes in particular has come under fire. The UK genetic watchdog GeneWatch states that apart from in specific cases (such as 'single gene' disorders), unidentified data variables, whether environmental or genetic, mean that modelling for predictive purposes produces meaningless results. According to GeneWatch director Helen Wallace, embedded assumptions in the 'bell curve' maths model lead to built-in flaws; for example, specifically in relation to the predictability of common complex/multifactorial disease. In a recent medical paper, she states that

> The results show that the potential for reducing the incidence of common diseases using environmental interventions targeted by genotype may be limited, except in special cases … The results therefore highlight the possibility – previously rejected on the basis of twin study results – that inherited genetic variants are important in determining risk only for the relatively rare familial forms of diseases such as breast cancer.
>
> (Wallace 2006)

Policy and regulation

A UK academic project, 'Governing Genetic Databases' states that 'There is no one piece of legislation that relates specifically to human genetic databases in England and Wales' (Ethox 2005). The Human Tissue Act, 2004 and the Data Protection Act, 1998 do however provide some important legal benchmarks for the governance of DNA databases and biobanks (the regulation of NDNAD is discussed further in Section two). Some other important regulatory benchmarks include the moratorium on the use of genetic information for insurance and 'best practice' guidelines accruing to genetic counselling (chapter 5).

The overall policy vacuum is especially significant given the need to identify and assess various risks and benefits in different contexts, processes that lie at the core of regulation and governance. A key example are the concerns about, for example, patient safeguards and privacy, balanced with potential benefits of data-sharing between research projects (GeneWatch 2009b). 'Guidelines' do exist in the form of recommendations from 'expert stakeholders', in documents drawn up by regulatory advisory bodies such as the Human Genetics Commission (HGC), Nuffield Council on Bioethics (NCoB), the UK National Screening Committee and international bodies such as the Human Genome Organisation (HUGO). Thus, each individual project will design its own ethical criteria, but there is no standardisation by type and accruing regulatory benchmark standard-setting. The UK Biobank Ethics and Governance Council is aiming to fill this particular governance gap with 'best practice' guidelines for the UK Biobank. Significantly, both Wellcome and NDNAD have been constructing regulatory frameworks governing the use and remit of biobanks and databases only after the banks have been set up. Similarly the UK stem cell bank is also constructing regulatory 'best practice' (chapter 2).

The regulatory scene thus consists of a range of institutions, some of which are directly responsible for policy, and others having more of an advisory role, with strong links to policy. Key advisory bodies are: NCoB, which reported on behavioural genetics in 2002 (NCoB 2002), and ran consultations on the NDNAD in 2006 (NCoB 2006); the UK Biobank Ethics and Governance Council, which oversees the Wellcome Biobank, HGC, the Genetics and Insurance Committee (GIAC), specific parliamentary select committees such as the Science and Technology committee, and so on.

The UK Biobank case study in Section two provides examples of the 'hybrid assemblages' which occur between governance and medical science in particular. Medical councils such as the Medical Research Council (MRC) are not simply 'expert stakeholders' asked to contribute to governance; to an extent, they *are* governance, and simultaneously stakeholders. Such blurring occurs because a relatively small pool of 'key stakeholders' sit on different committees and have 'strong ties' links to each other. Scientists and medical practitioners in many contexts, including in regulatory contexts, are commenting on biobanks and databases. Examples include cancer research units, bio-infomatics research units such as Sanger, third world epidemiologists, and genetic counsellors (Clarke 1998). Civil society/public engagement with regulation tends to consist of specific 'experts' and stakeholders (NGOs, patient groups, bio-ethics experts, academics, and so on), who contribute to governance through interaction with bodies such as NCoB and the Science and Technology Select Committee.

EU legislation informs the UK regulatory picture, although the UK does set its own legal framework. The EU 2004 Tissues and Cells directive (CEC 2004) provided an important overview of the regulatory and ethical issues at stake in the storage and use of human bio-material. The UK has also had to take legal notice of the recent EU human rights ruling on NDNAD samples (Section 2). The Council of Europe's convention on human rights and bio-medicine, which the UK has not signed, governs genetic research and discrimination and also has a protocol on gene test regulation (Wallace 2008b).

Global/international governance advisory bodies such as HUGO and Human Proteome Organisation have discussed health priorities, and ethical issues such as benefit sharing, and the Organisation for Economic Cooperation and Development (OECD) has also addressed this topic (OECD 2008), as has the World Health Organisation (WHO 2005). UNESCO has also made statements on the storage and use of genetic data (UNESCO 2002). International stakeholders are stepping into regulatory voids and co-constructing self-defined 'best practice' (Mayrhofer and Prainsack 2009), such as the ISSCR (chapter 2).

Section two: case studies of the UK Biobank and the National DNA Database (NDNAD)

This section provides narratives of the UK biobank and NDNAD, showing how the means, the aims and objectives, and the risks and benefits of these biobanks/databases are framed by different prime movers.

Case study 1: UK Biobank

The UK biobank aims to link individuals' genetic information with some lifestyle and other personal data and medical information, age, sex, post code, etc. The belief is that all the information may help in identifying variable interactions between genes, the environment, lifestyle and other factors, thus informing research on multifactoral (common complex) diseases, including predicting disease. The Wellcome Trust has enlisted substantial government and policy support for its biobank. This hybrid convergence between government and non-government, public and private, is characteristic of the types of mergers between public, private, and the spaces in between, happening across various sectors of bioscience, and is a familiar theme in the governance of human genetics as this book demonstrates. A new ethics committee, the UK Biobank Ethics and Governance Council, was set up to monitor the UK Biobank (EGC 2007). This is an 'independent' body, funded by the Wellcome Trust and the MRC.

A letter sent out to recruit donors for the biobank in 2008 provides a useful narrative:

> We are writing to ask for your help in studying the prevention and treatment of cancer, heart attacks, strokes, diabetes, dementia, joint problems, and many other serious diseases. This medical research project, called "UK Biobank", will involve 500,000 people aged 40–69 from all around the UK. Taking part is not intended to help you directly, but it should give future generations a much better chance of living their lives free of diseases that disable and kill.
>
> UK Biobank has been set up by the Department of Health, Medical Research Council and Scottish Executive, and by the Wellcome Trust medical charity. It is also supported by the Welsh Assembly Government,

by health research charities (such as the British Heart Foundation and Cancer Research UK) and by the National Health Service. People to invite are being identified from contact details in NHS records (without access to any medical information) which have been processed in confidence on behalf of the NHS.

(UK Biobank 2008)

An alternative biobank narrative from a Watchdog campaigner is less positive:

the decision to start the biobank was taken by so few people ... suddenly you've got a flagship genetic research project, which none of the geneticists think is going to work ... Most genetic epidemiologists are [critical] ... some of them have spoken out.

('Jenny')

'Jenny's' response shows clearly that means and ends are contested territory, as the following sub-section explores in more detail.

The stated aim of the UK Biobank is disease prevention, treatment and cure, through diagnostic and predictive usage of DNA samples. GeneWatch provides the following outline of the UK Biobank:

The aim of Biobank UK is to identify the genetic and environmental factors predisposing individuals to common diseases such as heart disease, cancer and mental illness ... The MRC states that this understanding would be used to predict the likelihood that an individual would develop a disease so that medicines could be used to prevent its onset rather than as a treatment for symptoms once a disease develops.

(GeneWatch 2002)

The aims of the Biobank were also described by 'Ian':

what UK Biobank is interested in is, you get the sample, you then do analysed, [and] randomised samples testing ... and link this with longer term health records ... picking out trends, picking out ... patterns.

('Ian')

Many patient groups are extremely supportive of the use of the UK Biobank as a means to an end – the treatment and cure of diseases. This includes the case study patient groups People's Voice for Medical Advance, the 'pro genetics' patient lobby group Genetic Interest Group, and the Association of Medical Research Charities. Support also comes from 'independent' patients such as those framing themselves (for example, in online communities) as part of 'genetic communities' of different types. However patient responses are complex, existing on a spectrum from 'pro research' patient groups, to Disability Rights groups who generally focus on risk frames relating to the end uses of genetic information (chapter 5). While patient groups and charities are generally supportive of end uses of future medical applications, some are ambivalent, not to say critical, about 'non-medical' uses of bio-information and issues such as privacy (see NDNAD). This ambivalence represents an important crossover point between patient groups and genetic watchdogs.

Many of the diseases named are multifactorial; that is, they are 'common complex' diseases with multiple causalities, many of which are unknown. 'Jenny' argues that the stated goal of the UK Biobank – to tackle multifactorial disease – is so broad as to be unviable. This is especially so when it is compared with smaller, targeted biobank and genetic databases attached to specific diseases known to have strong genetic links.

> the idea that you could add the genes into risk assessment and then be able to tell if you were going to get it [a specific disease], and who wasn't ... from a scientific point of view I was sceptical.
>
> ('Jenny')

Genetic watchdogs such as GeneWatch are also particularly sceptical about the predictive function of the UK Biobank, and about how environmental information, for example, will actually be used in tandem with genetic information to accurately predict predisposition to disease. This approach to disease prevention is highly controversial. Many scientists believe that prediction of future common illnesses by testing people's genetic make-up is unlikely to be a successful or cost-effective means of disease prevention (GeneWatch 2002).

This analysis has led to GeneWatch's describing predictive modelling as 'genetic horoscopes'.[7] The Wellcome Trust does state, however, that exploring genetic complexity and uncertainty, is an important research rationale: 'perhaps one of the outcomes [of Biobank] will be that it's impossible to predict [disease outcomes] because of interactions with the environment' (Robert Terry).[8] Uncertainty about aims and outcomes because of genetic complexity, and also the blurring over diagnostic or predictive methodologies, was also identified by 'Ian':

> if the techniques develop for data analysis over the next five, ten years, then I'm sure [the UK biobank will] see a lot more [disease, condition] susceptibility genes identified. But how you actually use that information ... in a diagnostic or therapeutic way ... remains to be seen ... given the muddiness of complex disease, I mean, 10 years ago it was thought that we'd know a hell of a lot more now than we actually do or are even close to understanding in terms of complexity so it's sort of wait and see if something comes up
>
> ('Ian')

Chapter 6 identifies how many people are asking the question: Are we concentrating on genetic aspects of illness at the expense of others? This is also being asked in relation to the UK Biobank. Common complex disorders are not the same as 'single gene' disorders; they are affected by many variables. Watchdogs say that geneticisation means that health is constructed in terms of individuals being continually susceptible to being in a disease state, and that this has major implications for policy. GeneWatch has specifically critiqued the remit of the UK Biobank in relation to health policy, relating this to issues of social justice. Not only is the viability of the genetic information seen as questionable, but the potential to individualise health responsibility and not address wider contextual issues of poverty and environment are key concerns. These issues are returned to in chapter 6.

There are hopes, both from those critical and those supportive of the UK Biobank, that epidemiology-led studies may provide some openings for social and environmental justice interventions to be pursued through policy, as genetic complexity identifies environmental variables (Prainsack *et al.* 2008). These hopes are undercut by very real concerns that genetic information could actually be used to further undermine sustainable development policy aims and agendas, through focusing on 'genetic susceptibility' and thus individualising health risks and responsibilities; see Di Chiro (2004a, 2008) and further discussion in chapters 4, 6.

Frames of 'future promise' (see chapter 8) are consistently invoked in relation to disease prevention and cure. The promissory framing of the biobank by Wellcome is also a common scientific, regulatory account of the biobank.

There is a linked framing of 'public good', invocations of citizenship and altruism (chapter 6):

> Improving the health of future generations ... Do you want to do something good today? Not just for yourself, but for our children and our children's children?
>
> (UK Biobank 2007a)

Wellcome frames the donation of DNA in a similar way to the donation of blood, or organs; chapter 2 identified a similar use of 'public good' discourse in relation to egg donation. There is also a taken-for-granted assumption in the Wellcome 'public good' discourse, that whilst not necessarily benefiting specific donors, public benefits will be felt by *all* members of 'future generations'. However, other prime movers feel that this is unlikely to be the case. Western societies are far more likely to benefit from products such as drugs accruing from biobanks, than are any third world sample donors, without a health care infrastructure, which is why bodies such as WHO are focusing on benefit sharing as a third world health outcome. However even within the UK, there are extreme differences between health authorities in relation to what patients can expect in the form of available treatments. These are not evenly distributed amongst UK publics; there is a 'postcode lottery' in relation to healthcare (King's Fund 2008). It is also possible that people pre-disposed to genetic conditions may further lose out in terms of public healthcare availability.

The following sub-sections set out other issues arising from the UK Bio-bank which are being debated by different publics. First, public concerns have been raised about the ownership[9] of publicly donated bio-material:

> I give my data in good faith to ... a public project. And my data could get used by companies ... to make profits.
>
> ('Alice')

It remains unclear what the protocol for patenting and profiting from publicly donated DNA is, in relation to the UK Biobank, whose policies were still in draft form in 2009.[10] The spectacular variety of public and privately owned biobanks and databases means that different contexts and criteria inform the specifics of use and ownership. This is particularly true of privately owned databases of publicly donated bio-material, of which the Icelandic database is a well known example. ETC talks about 'enclosures' and 'biopiracy' (ETC 2008b) in relation to privately held databases of the samples of populations, and indigenous peoples' samples (Prainsack *et al.* 2008; Harry *et al.* 2000; Howard 2001). 'Watchdogs', environmental and anti globalisation activists, and indigenous campaign groups such as the Indigenous Peoples Council have raised concerns about the inequities involved when an indigenous popu-lation or disease community provides (sometimes unknowingly) the resources for a private database owned by 'big pharma' (Chan and de Wildt 2007). Intellectual property is discussed further in chapter 4.

The concept of benefit sharing (Schroeder 2007) has been developed as a response to these concerns, by bio-ethical institutions such as HUGO with the capacity to advocate 'best practice' internationally across private and public settings, in the form of advice and 'guidelines'. This has been seen as an important move towards the mitigation of identified risks and injustices in relation to access and equity. A key issue has been the identified discrepancy between those providing the sample, and the ownership of the biobank/ database itself and the ownership and equitable distribution of benefits – [bio] resources – such as drugs. 'Benefit sharing' aims to address these issues.

The picture is again complicated by the different types and remits of bio-bank models; for example, 'best practice' guidelines can only inform those involved in private databases and are not enforceable. Different protocols may be applicable, and also more enforceable, for publicly funded databases. 'Benefit sharing' amongst donors and public stakeholders in the context of the UK Biobank is generally framed in terms of future public health out-comes. Concerns about how, where and under what circumstances commer-cial use of public data is siphoned off for private profit have also been raised by civil society groups. Bio-ethics debates are moving to address to discuss 'community' benefit sharing (Chadwick 2005). But which community should benefit and in what context? For example, a 'disease community', a local indigenous population, national population, global population, are all different sorts of communities. Also, there are problems about what counts as a benefit; benefit sharing as a bio-ethics discourse primarily relates to equitable access to the end products – drugs, for example. However there are other potential end uses which are more disputed benefits. For example, some Disability Rights activists contest the idea that more prenatal screening accruing from use of biobank/database information, followed by termination of pregnancies, counts as a benefit per se. Some in fact frame this as a risk (the eugenic 'slippery slope'; chapter 5). Further, the viability of trickle-down benefits is disputed in many contexts; for example, 'postcode lotteries' of access to medical treatments in the UK will affect who benefits in the future.

Chapter 7 discusses informed consent in detail. Informed consent has been a controversial issue in relation to the terms under which material has been taken for privately owned biobanks/databases, and this has led to the development of informed consent debates in this arena. In the case of the UK Biobank, donors would not be given feedback about their own 'genetic information', and their data would be anonymised for large-scale modelling use. In this case, the ethics of informed consent does not relate specifically to risks accruing to the feeding back of information to the donor, as it might in relation to another biobank – for example a biobank of specific samples accruing to a specific disease. Whether people should have the option of having this information (if, for example's sake, specific single gene information was found to have an important bearing on an individual donor's potential health outcomes) has been a subject of ethical debate for Wellcome/the UK Biobank, though the current edition of the UK Biobank's Ethics and Governance Framework makes no mention of feedback to donors (UK Biobank 2007).

In relation to potential future uses of genetic information, uncertainty about the 'secondary use' of database/biobank information is a key sticking point for informed consent protocols, such as its use for genetic testing and screening (chapter 5). 'Broad consent' as used by UK Biobank and others remains contentious: it is contrary to the Helsinki Declaration[11] which requires people to be informed of who is doing the research and any conflicts of interest. Generally, the different aims of the different typologies of biobanks necessitate different models of 'informed consent' from the person whose biological sample is being taken, although there will be some commonalities. Standardisation may also be relevant and may be legally necessary (see chapter 7). The process of drawing up and administering regulation would necessitate a great deal of administration and resourcing.

The terms and conditions of the UK Biobank are likely to protect individuals from the potential use of genetic information by other third parties, but the issue of discrimination has long been identified as an important issue in respect of sample use. Here again the issue of blurring medical and non-medical use is key; a medical sample could be used in a non-medical context or for a non-medical outcome. When UK genetics and civil liberties watchdogs and campaign groups voice concerns about 'genetic underclasses', the key concern is that an individual's genetic information will be used to discriminate against them in a variety of contexts, such as school, the work-place, insurance and mortgages, and healthcare. There is a potential that individuals will be discriminated against or stigmatised because of bio-infor-mation which is known about them in these specific contexts, which has been acquired from bio-databases. The implications of genetic discrimination have enrolled a broad set of stakeholders highly alert to these issues; the Consumer Association, trades unions, watchdogs concerned with racial discrimination, and also, interestingly, generally 'pro genetic' patient groups. Such concerns have also been identified by regulatory frameworks in the UK, for example, such as the HGC and GIAC. Such concerns and caveats can be summarised as:

• Being unfair per se (people can't help being winners and losers in a genetic lottery).
• Being likely to be wrong or uncertain – limits of predictability except in specific cases.
• Framing out other variables equally or more important, such as environ-mental impacts.
• Placing responsibility/agency on the individual, not society. The 'indivi-dualising' of responsibility is seen as a major issue of social justice (chapter 6).
• Having potential human rights implications in terms of privacy breaches and genetic discrimination.

If an individual's genetic information is known, this could affect their work chances, or their compensation claims in certain circumstances; if it was known that they had a specific 'gene for' susceptibility to different types of pollution, for example (GeneWatch 2009d). There is also a risk that genetic information will be used to 'blame and frame' people as being 'genetically predisposed' to be susceptible to pollution. This is a social justice issue in that it individualises responsibility while detracting attention away from causalities (Di Chiro 2008). These concerns were expressed by 'Jenny' who discussed how specific companies were conducting research into genetic susceptibility:

> why are these companies so interested in [genetic susceptibility to pollu-tion], is it because they want to blame the genes. Rather than do some-thing about ... emissions.
>
> ('Jenny')

Since 2002 there has been a UK moratorium on the use of genetic informa-tion for insurance purposes; this moratorium is a 'concordat' developed by the Department of Health; advisory governance bodies (GIAC and the HGC); the Association of British Insurers; and other stakeholders such as patient groups (Dept of Health and ABI 2005). The moratorium has been extended until 2014. This is one of the few arenas where a 'strong' use of the precautionary principle (Ahteensuu 2004) is in operation. The concordat states: 'very few tests can predict with any certainty when an illness might begin, or how severe it might be'. Bio-ethicist Professor Soren Holm has advocated the use of genetic information for insurance purposes (BMJ 2007). His key argument is that there is currently an [illogical] distinction being made, between the use of genetic and non-genetic information in terms of risk prediction/assessment for insurance. The example he gives, is that having a high body mass index (being fat) is information already used for insurance [risk] assessment, for predictive purposes. Holm raises the important issue of 'genetic exceptionalism' (chapter 6); is there something so 'different' about genetic information that it warrants special circumstances? However, many argue that genetics should be a 'special case'. First, there is potential for unfair risk assessment based on over-reliance on questionable genetic modelling. Thus one *could* in fact say, in this specific case, that genetic information *is* different to being fat, in terms of a predictor of risk susceptibility. Second, there might be unfair access to, and use of, this information by others (employers, mortgage lenders, health service) and so extra protection is needed for individuals. Civil society stakeholders have been very active in lobbying for a moratorium on social justice grounds.

> when the insurance industry says: right, we know your genes, therefore we're going to give you a higher premium … there's a major injustice question there … Based on … using limited knowledge for certain ends.
>
> ('Andrew')

Risk is discussed further in chapter 8.

Case study 2: the UK[12] National DNA Database (NDNAD).

Sometimes also referred to as the police DNA database, or the 'forensic' DNA database, the NDNAD is a database of individuals' DNA profiles. Ministers also stated in 2006 that on the NDNAD [in 2004] '12,095 volunteer records were loaded. … Between 1 April 2005 and 10 January 2006, a further 3,221 volunteer profiles have been loaded' (Hansard 2006a). Samples from most operational police personnel are also held on a related database, the Police Elimination Database, as hairs or skin cells from investigating police officers would also be left at the scene of a crime. DNA samples have been used by the police in a limited form since 1984 (GeneWatch 2009d). The NDNAD was set up in 1995. In 2001, an extension of the 1984 Police and Criminal Evidence Act (PACE) allowed all DNA samples taken from individuals held in police custody to be retained indefinitely, irrespective of whether individuals were later acquitted (GeneWatch 2009d). The 2001 law required the individual to be charged with a recordable offence. There was a second important change in the law in 2003 (which came into force in 2004) which allowed DNA to be taken on arrest (rather than charge).

Samples are obtained from crime scenes, or taken from individuals whilst held in police custody. The DNA profiles of children as young as ten are now held on the NDNAD. The government took control of the database from the Forensic Science Service in December 2005; a Home Office unit is responsible for regulating the database (NPIA 2007). Proposed changes to PACE outlined in the Home Office consultation (2007a) infer a legal shift in the proposed use of NDNAD; namely the use of NDNAD for identifying individuals, not finding DNA matches for specific crimes (GeneWatch 2007).

Box 3.2

Some facts and figures

*   The NDNAD cost £300 million during 2002–7.[13]

*   According to the Home Office in 2006, the database held samples of 5.2% of the UK population (3.1 million individuals),[14] compared with an EU average of 1.13%.[15]

*   On 1 December 2005, there were 24,168 persons under 18 on the NDNAD who had not been charged or cautioned for any offence.[16]

*   3 in 4 black men aged 15–34 are now on the NDNAD.[17]

DNA profiles/samples are one of a number of types of 'biometric information', such as fingerprints and iris scans, 'used to confirm or disprove an individual's suspected involvement in a criminal offence and to establish identity' (Home Office 2007a, Section 3.32). The digital record of the DNA profile information contained within the DNA sample itself, and/or the physical DNA sample itself – the law is unclear, circumstances vary, according to the HGC (2002)[18] – is kept on the NDNAD. The police are able to search the NDNAD to find DNA profile matches.

The Home Office and the Association of Chief Police Officers state that NDNAD's purpose is solving crime. The primary use of the NDNAD is forensic: identifying individuals through their DNA profile, and finding matches for DNA profiles already held on the NDNAD, to DNA found at crime scenes. According to the Home Office,

'The national DNA database is a key police intelligence tool that helps to:

- quickly identify offenders
- make earlier arrests
- secure more convictions
- provide critical investigative leads for police investigations' (NPIA 2007).

Such forensic use of DNA samples/profiles also includes the identification of bodies, for example following major disasters.

Reports by the HGC (2002) and by the House of Lords Science and Technology committee (HL 2005) both strongly recommended that an independent ethics committee for the NDNAD be established urgently; an independent Ethics Advisory Group met for the first time on 3 September 2007 (NDNAD EG 2008). Neither the Human Tissue Act (Dept of Health 2004b) which governs research on other DNA databases and biobanks, or the Data Protection Act (DCA 1998), cover the NDNAD; rather, there are specific exemptions from these Acts relating to the collection and use of DNA for 'purposes relating to the prevention and detection of crime'.

In a landmark ruling, judges at the European Court of Human Rights in December 2008 endorsed the recommendations of the Nuffield Council on Bioethics against storing DNA profiles and samples of innocent people on the National DNA Database (ECHR 2008). The Court of seventeen judges unanimously ruled that keeping the samples and fingerprints of two UK men, who had been arrested but never convicted of any crime, constituted a breach of their human rights.[19] The judgment was based solely on a violation of Article 8 – the right to respect for a private life. In response to this ruling, the UK Home Secretary announced the publication of a white paper on forensics in 2009, with the aim of creating a more proportionate and effective system of retention. The government has also announced the immediate withdrawal of samples from children aged under ten years from the database (around seventy samples) (HC Library 2009).

As with the UK Biobank, civil society concerns refer to the means (the terms and conditions) in which data is collated and stored, the stated aims and objectives, and other consequences. Examples of key issues and the ways in which they are being framed by different publics are given below.

The forensic use of DNA samples, used in conjunction with good, well resourced policing, clearly helps to solve crime. But it is unclear how many crimes are solved *solely* by relying on DNA, such as Operation Advance (Home Office 2007b). Further, there is a great deal of difference between forensic and predictive use of sample data. Some have identified a 'usage creep' of NDNAD from forensic use (solving existing crime) to predictive use (predicting future criminality) embedded in the 2007 PACE review. Everyone on the NDNAD is treated as a member of a 'risky' population as a result of having been arrested (i.e. is assumed to be at risk of committing a future offence).

It is questionable whether a DNA profile alone can predict that someone is or is likely to become a criminal. Criminality is not a genetic 'fact'; it is a social, political and legal construct. This is a key non-medical example of concerns about 'geneticisation' (chapter 6), which might be summed up by asking whether someone can be 'genetically predisposed' to crime, to which the straightforward answer is no. Whilst 'Fragile X' (NCoB 2002) does have a strong genetic link to 'anti social behaviour', it is a unique case and is still multi factoral. Many ask, in terms of crime prevention specifically, how useful the NDNAD is relative to, for example, other measures addressing social exclusion and poverty.

The predictive use of samples is especially relevant to the use of samples from innocent people and minor offenders, the subject of the landmark 2008 ruling. During the research timeframe, a range of prime movers including governance sources such as NCoB and the HGC[20] voiced concerns:

> With regard to predictive testing, we concluded that neither genetic nor non genetic information should be used to predict future behaviour with a view to detaining an individual who has not been convicted of a crime.
>
> (NCoB 2002)

NCoB launched a public consultation on NDNAD in November 2006 (NCoB 2006) and concluded (September 2007) that DNA of innocent people should not be kept by police, amongst other recommendations (NCoB 2007). During 2003–7, the fact that samples taken from innocent people and those convicted of minor offences are kept on the police database attracted much public criticism. GeneWatch argued that:

> time limits on how long individuals can be retained on the DNA Database should be reintroduced – so that only people convicted of serious crimes have their records retained permanently.
>
> (GeneWatch *et al.* 2007)

The civil liberties NGO Liberty, a UK children's rights organisation (ARCH), and the genetic watchdog GeneWatch stated in a 2007 briefing that:

> Expanding the number of individuals on the National DNA Database is unlikely to be a cost-effective way to tackle crime. Only a tiny proportion of crimes are solved using DNA ... There is no evidence that keeping innocent people on the Database for life solves more crimes.
>
> (GeneWatch *et al.* 2007)

Significantly in the light of the 2008 ruling, many framed their concerns in terms of civil liberties and human rights: 'If you're not convicted your DNA should be destroyed just on the grounds of human rights'(BBC 2006a[21]). The NDNAD has received much national mass-media attention, for example over the issue of children's samples held on the register (Hansard 2006b, *Independent* 2006). Many media stories about the NDNAD have been 'success stories' about the forensic use of DNA in solving old murder cases. The 2008 human rights ruling on the storage of DNA samples was also a big story because a legal precedent has now been set. This may change future media reportage in terms of how the efficacy of DNA in predictive crime solving is presented.

The watchdogs Liberty and GeneWatch, and the Nuffield Council on Bio-ethics have all raised concerns that NDNAD will exacerbate or reproduce existing 'institutionalised' discrimination in a number of contexts.[22] Examples of potential discrimination include racial discrimination:

Example 1

> The government should look into why black people are over-represented on the UK's DNA database, says a black police officers' group. National Black Police Association spokesman Keith Jarrett ... said an inquiry should examine if officers used the 'same robustness' in taking samples from different groups.
>
> (NBPA 2006)

Example 2

> the Home Office has given permission for a controversial genetic study to be undertaken using the DNA samples on the police database to see if it is possible to predict a suspect's ethnic background or skin colour from them. Permission has been given for the DNA being collected on the police database to be used in 20 research studies.
>
> (*Observer* 2006)

The specifics of potential discrimination in relation to subsets of the general population reflect a broader public concern about genetic discrimination in both medical and non-medical contexts, as discussed in relation to the UK Biobank. Thus issues of discrimination in particular blur between medical and 'non-medical' uses and remits of different databases including the NDNAD. Some other examples cited by campaigners and by regulators include children having their 'cards marked for life', for example, by being 'genetically predisposed to anti social behaviour'. The 2002 Nuffield report was strongly opposed to genetic research on anti social behaviour. However the tendency to 'medicalise' childhood behavioural problems is a growing one; with large numbers of children in the US and UK diagnosed with the attention deficit disorder ADHD and treated with drugs (NetDoctor ca: 2008). Another example is the use of medical databases to extract (political, personal) information by third parties; for example, police access to medical databases (*Computer Weekly* 2008).

> A private firm has secretly been keeping the genetic samples and personal details of hundreds of thousands of arrested people. Police forces use the company LGC to analyse DNA samples taken from people they arrest ... the firm has kept copies, together with highly personal demographic details of the individuals including their names, ages, skin colour and addresses.
>
> (*Observer* 2006)

This startling 2006 news story flags public concerns about the use of genetic information: what information could be obtained from a sample (or profile?), with what implications? Who has access to the NDNAD? Who 'owns' the information? GeneWatch is concerned about:

> the erosion of people's privacy. For example, partial matches with DNA profiles on the National DNA Database can reveal who a person is related to (including paternity and non-paternity).
>
> (GeneWatch 2008)

The NDNAD has catalysed the emergence of a number of autonomous public campaign groups across the political spectrum:

> We believe [the NDNAD] ... is an unjustified accumulation of private data by the State, which erodes the presumption of innocence and feeds a culture of authoritarianism.
>
> (E-Petition 2007)

Libertarian groups such as Progress Educational Trust (PET) have also voiced concerns. In this specific context, they have framed the issue of the risks associated with the police database in a similar way to that of civil liberty groups and watchdogs such as GeneWatch. Here is the publicity for a PET event in 2005: 'Do the genetic databases used by the police help them solve more common crimes or do they threaten our civil liberties?' (PET 2007) Significantly, GeneWatch was invited by PET to speak at this event. PET often disagrees with civil liberties groups and genetic watchdogs over the 'medical' potential of DNA databases.

The issues of privacy and civil liberties are raised by public groups in relation to all types of biobanks and databases, whether medical or non-medical. Key to all concerns about privacy and civil liberties in relation to biobanks and databases is the lack of coherence, the lack of safeguards, and the 'wild west frontier' aspect of such issues:

> my data might have gone to insurance companies or who knows where it could go ... there isn't a proper relationship of trust between me and the people who've got my data.
>
> ('Alice')

Trust is a key theme here, and many public concerns relate to a lack of trust. Bio-surveillance concerns can be defined as the use of bioinfomatic data (iris scans, genetic profiles, fingerprints) by the state or third parties to collate information about members of the public. Such concerns are invoked by campaigners against a background picture of a political climate where civil liberties have declined through legal amendments throughout the New Labour era and particularly 'post 9/11'; for example the 42-day ruling

(*Independent* 2008), which has seen many Establishment figures (Liberty 2008) make very strident comments about loss of civil liberties. The concerns about privacy and civil liberties infringements in relation to bio-surveillance link to debates about ID cards (NO2ID 2008), and to concerns about military bio-surveillance (Altmann 2004). These are issues about access to bio-information (who has it? who would use it and how?) and trust; where and in what are 'the public' supposed to put their trust? There are concerns that state bio-surveillance strategies may use and/or create biobanks and databases as sources of bio-information, for example Home Office research on samples from the NDNAD.

Conclusion

This chapter has shown that there are many different types of biobanks and databases and that there is both confusion and lack of regulation in relation to typologies, means and ends. Even relatively well regulated biobanks like the UK Biobank have significant gaps relating to who owns the data and who might financially benefit from patents accruing from publicly dona-ted samples. The chapter has identified that there is blurring between medical and non-medical uses and/or outcomes, of biobanks and databases. Databases set up for one purpose (e.g. crime, health or research purposes) can be used for the other(s). The 'governance gaps' which exist in relation to biobanks and databases are likely to generate further public engagement and debate, for example over issues of informed consent, benefit sharing and discrimination.

The chapter provided case study narrative detail about the UK Biobank, a 'medical' biobank, and the NDNAD, a 'non-medical' one, outlining key issues framed by different publics such as disease and crime prevention. For example, it has provided a narrative of opposition to the storage and use of the DNA samples of innocent people on the NDNAD, an issue which emerged as a key moment of public debate on several occasions, culminating in the 2008 Human Rights ruling. Importantly, while context-specific risks and benefits are outlined by these different publics in relation to the two case studies, there are a number of issues which blur boundaries because their implications 'leak' from one site to another. For example, the *predictive* use of genetic information is a common concern, whether medical (health) or non-medical (crime). This relates both to the viability of the bio-information (whether this predictive use is scientifically accurate or whether it is simply a 'genetic horoscope') and the social justice and civil liberties implications of this predictive use in many contexts. Predictive functions could 'blame and frame' individuals for their genetic makeup and detract attention away from envir-onmental social justice interventions such as poverty alleviation. Genetic dis-crimination is also a common concern across medical and non-medical sites, exacerbated by the potential for information taken in one context to be used in another.

The framing of the public debates is also itself the subject of critique by certain prime movers. For example, the UK Biobank frames its remit in relation to disease prevention. Mobilising public support for broad public health outcomes is different to mobilising public support for targeting specific diseases, but the two issues – preventing specific diseases, and achieving population health – are somewhat confused in 'official' promissory accounts. The publicly accessible literature for the UK Biobank mobilises a discourse of prevention and potential treatments and cures for diseases which affect large sectors of the population. This framing also sets up a sense that to support the biobank is to be 'pro health' and a 'good citizen'. Other prime movers have wished to discuss a broader agenda of what public health consists of and how it should be achieved, voicing concerns that the UK Biobank reflects a geneticised account of health policy, rather than a social justice-orientated one, which predominates in policy discourse. These are familiar themes of public engagement, power relations and stakes-setting which run throughout the book. Framing broader debates about what constitutes 'public good and public health' and what strategies are appropriate, may contribute to finding convergence points, 'crosstalk' (Bucchi 2004), between civil society perspectives.

This chapter identified that developments in sequencing have significantly impacted on the typologies and remits of different biobanks and databases. The following chapter provides a more detailed narrative of how databases /biobanks of bio-information and samples are being utilised, using the example of pharmacogenetics/omics ('pharmacoG'). In providing this narrative, chapter 4 focuses attention on the economic drivers – increasingly referred to as 'the bio-economy'– which are arguably pushing the pharmacoG agenda, and discusses related issues of ownership which have also been touched on in this chapter.

4 'PharmacoG' as product and process

Introduction

This chapter defines 'pharmacoG' (a combined term for both pharmacogenomics and pharmocogenetics), providing in Section one a narrative of the science and the associated products and promises. 'PharmacoG' is defined as a 'hybrid' techno-science involving many different publics including assemblages of governance, science and industry. Section two introduces the 'bio-economy', namely the economic framework within which pharmacoG is evolving, focusing on how concepts and emergent issues are being framed, and engaged with, by civil society prime movers. While some prime movers such as patient groups are happy to support 'big pharma' in their quest for pharmacoG-related cures, others are voicing concerns over issues such as access, ownership (intellectual property) and identity. A range of prime movers are identifying how the bio-economic agenda impacts not only on product development and delivery, but on the setting of global health agendas.

Section one: a pharmacoG narrative

Medical science is now interested to understand how the function and expression of a specific gene, or set of genes, which code for the creation of useful proteins in the body, can play a role in the manifestation of a specific disease or condition.[1] The use of drugs to regulate gene expression is the field of pharmacogenetics/omics. The terminology is fuzzy, even within the scientific community:

> even though everybody has a gut feeling of what [pharmacogenomics] means, a clear-cut definition is still lacking. Thus, although most agree that pharmacogenomics has something to do with the whole genome and is therefore more comprehensive than pharmocogenetics, these terms are used interchangeably and for the same purpose by many.
>
> (Lackner 2002)

This comment from 2002 is still relevant today and hence this chapter uses the term 'pharmacoG' incorporating the 'etics and omics' suffixes. Pharmaco *genetics* is a term to discuss drugs relating to a specific gene/set of genes. Pharmaco*genomics* is framed by some as a more exact, fast-tracked and cohesive means of identifying relevant gene sequences, via the use of genetic information contained in the entire genome, to understand disease and trait expression, and to provide potential products. A consistently expressed goal of pharmacogenomics is the production of drugs aimed at a particular individual's genomic expression, and/or the specifically differentiated genetic expression of a specific form of a disease or condition such as a specific type of cancer; this is so-called 'personalised pharmaco' (Evans *et al.* 1999), as 'Alice' explains:

> there are lots of advances in prognosis and diagnosis. If I've got leukaemia, people can look at the expression profiles of my genes, so which genes are being expressed and which genes aren't being ... I could be diagnosed as having type A which means I'm going to respond to this kind of chemotherapy
>
> ('Alice')

'PharmacoG' is not only the term for the end product (drugs): it enrols the sense of process; namely, that 'pharmacoG' is intrinsically connected to the DNA sequencing process. During 2003–7, rapid developments in the technologies used to sequence DNA dramatically speeded up the process by which genetic information is sequenced or 'read'. Sequencing DNA involves both physical data sequencing (for example through mass spectrometry)[2] and computer analysis of this data (bioinfomatics). Bioinfomatics has been defined as 'the use of computers to store, search and characterize the genetic code of genes, the proteins linked to each gene and their associated functions'.[3] An important development within bioinfomatics has been the ability to rapidly identify Single Nucleotide Polymers (SNPs) as a means of 'marking' or identifying genetic/genomic variation.[4] The accuracy of sequencing and mapping techniques is challenged by genetic watchdogs, in terms of the veracity of claims to be able to 'map' genomes; for example, what the information contained in a DNA sequence actually signifies, how much of a specific genome is actually being 'mapped', and finally whether this 'mapping' amounts to reliable, replicable knowledge claims. GeneWatch, for example, has focused a great deal of attention on the disjuncture between promissory claims to have 'mapped'[5] genes and genomes and the lack of end products. Chapter 3 showed that GeneWatch identifies a number of specific problems with the claims being made for genetic and genomic testing in relation to disease expression and predictability, such as disagreements between scientists over what specific genetic variations actually signify; meanings are contested and hence outcomes – end products such as drugs – are uncertain.

Genes 'code for' proteins, and proteins are themselves now being sequenced; the field of proteomics (McNally and Glasner 2007). Proteomics may overtake genomics in both discursive and scientific terms:

in terms of finding disease genes ... I suspect that people will focus on protein-targeting ... there's going to be a lot more short-term mileage out of 'intelligent drug design' based on proteomics and improved protein structural modelling which can pick up the effects of those subtle differences.

(Online chat with scientist 2005)

Bioinfomatics, genetics, genomics and proteomics are thus all aspects of pharmacoG as a converged techno-scientific site which is both the field of study – the reading of the information and the inferring of meaning – and the site of application; specific products for a specific target. PharmacoG is thus another 'hybrid site', consisting of multiple types of processes and outcomes (applications), embedded in multiple linked actor networks and political spaces. Hence pharmacoG is not easily characterised; in fact this is a major talking point in the pharmacoG debate, and thus definitions are approached with caveats and caution.

Promises and products

PharmacoG's key 'future promise' discourse of better drug targeting has already been flagged above. However despite the huge promise of pharmacoG, there are currently very few pharmacoG-based treatments, let alone cures; there is a gap between the amount of investment at the R&D stage and the end result (Hopkins *et al.* 2007). This is despite the increase in genetic/ genomic information available: 'the gene for cystic fibrosis was found years ago and there's no cure for cystic fibrosis from that. CF is well defined as an illness ... and genomics hasn't led to a cure' ('Alice'). The 'future promise' of pharmacoG is a work in progress, and a highly contested one. It is likely that in some cases, pharmacoG will be able to identify which drugs *not* to give people, potentially meaning better targeting of existing drugs on specific population groups and the possibility of re-introducing drugs currently banned because of adverse effects on specific, perhaps now identifiable, population sub-groups.

> a lot of people have ... SARs or Severe Adverse Reactions to drugs ... in the US there's ... hundreds of thousands of deaths a year due to adverse effects to drugs. So one part of pharmaco genetics is [to] understand how drugs are metabolised ... identify[ing] genes that metabolise drugs and that's fairly well mapped out now.
>
> ('Ian')

Stem cell lines (chapter 2) are being identified by science and industry as potential sites for testing drugs; how will stem cell line A react to pharmaco product B? Thus bio-technological processes, such as the creation and use of human and animal tissues and cells, are intrinsically related to pharmacoG.

Animals are used in pharmacoG research processes in different ways for multiple functions. The 'lab rat' is no longer simply used to test the end product of a specific drug. Now, using a range of techniques including reproductive cloning, specific animals are produced to study the expression of a specific disease as well as to test the impacts of specific drugs, for example the creation of cloned mice carrying the CF gene (chapter 2). Animals have also been created as sources of potential end products, for example the 'Dolly' cloned sheep herd was created to express a specific human protein in their milk (*Independent* 1997). Such hybrids have profound ethical and philosophical significance (Haraway 1991). It is also significant that the animals are being created as the potential end product *of*, rather than simply the test site *for*, pharmacoG. This animal-based product delivery represents a particularly ambitious, and still highly experimental, manifestation of the field of 'edible vaccines'.[6] 'Big pharma' is thus moving into bio-tech, a move dictated at least in part by financial considerations, as ETC has noted:

> In light of the industry-wide drug development drought, Big Pharma is particularly attracted to companies with biotech products (referred to generally as 'biologics' because they are derived from living organisms rather than produced via chemistry) nearing regulatory approval.
>
> (ETC 2008: 26)

Nutrigenomics[7] and nutriceuticals[8] are specific types of pharmacoG-related products: they are 'smart foods', with smart marketing. Nutrigenomics is a means of harnessing genetic/genomic information for a new product context – the health/food supplement. Nutrigenomics promissory discourse focuses on the potential to help people 'eat right for their genotype/phenotype'; this incorporates both simple nutritional advice and also the potential for manufacturing genetic or other 'smart food' bio-products geared towards supplementing or helping the identified (genetic) problem.

Potential products are thus on a scale ranging from a health supplement as 'lifestyle choice' to the potential for vaccines, for example, to be processed through the human body by eating a bio-engineered product. Nutriceuticals are bio-engineered foods and supplements, defined on a blurred spectrum between a 'health food' and a drug, which claim to 'help' or 'supplement' a condition or problem, or claim to help in terms of preventing a potential condition; a genetically engineered version of current health foods such as live yoghurt drinks which claim to aid digestion.

Current trends include food giants such as Nestlé moving into genomic and nanotech research,[9] and a melding of food and pharmaco conglomerations. The vast investment from 'usual suspect' global mega-corporations such as Nestlé in this arena is suggestive of a trend into a perhaps more lucrative arena more likely to attract 'healthy rich, worried well' bio-consumers. There may be other reasons why there is a move into nutriceuticals. Carefully worded adverts could perhaps more easily pass advertising standards, enabling definitions of the effects of food supplements which necessitate less of a burden of 'proof' than standards for pharmaceutical products, along the lines of: 'this may help you metabolise your fat (as part of a healthy life-style ...)'. The move into neutriceuticals amongst 'big pharma' and food giants picks up on Eurobarometer data[10] which highlights that health is a core value for publics – and, importantly, such values can be developed commercially (Waldby 2002, Uusitalo 2008). Hence there is an interesting potential for a 'rebranding' of genetically modified products as 'health food', which may mean that the same publics who expressed concerns about health risks in relation to GM food might be persuaded to buy them if they are convinced that these products could provide health benefits.

Science and 'big pharma'; hybrid science

The scientific field is a particularly complex one, both in terms of defining the science and also in terms of 'who does what and where'. We have seen that many previously separate scientific disciplines are converging. Flagging this converging and shifting of disciplines in 2003, 'Alice' noted that 'it depends on whether you see bioinfomatics as a discipline in itself or just as a tool box that you can be trained in'. Everywhere, scientific disciplines are morphing into financial ventures. 'Ian' identifies this as 'translational' research:

> what I'd like to develop are stronger links with schools of pharmacy, schools of chemistry ... building those links so ... we've got translational research ... mov[ing] things down the development process, not only because it's interesting biologically, but ... adding [financial] value.
>
> ('Ian')

This movement between disciplines is thus catalysing structural changes within the modus operandi of 'big pharma'. This converged, translational research is influenced by economic imperatives and also associated political considerations, such as in which countries hES research is legally allowed. These hybrid narratives, driven as they are by political and economic imperatives as well as scientific and technical translational developments, are the result, and key examples of, what is increasingly being referred to the 'bio-economy' (Birch 2006), discussed in Section Two.

PharmacoG and bio-tech are melding both as the sites of scientific practice, and as industry 'assemblages', firstof all in the form of takeovers and mergers. According to ETC group, 'There were 23 pharma/biotech mergers and acquisitions in 2005; 24 deals in 2006; and 19 in 2007, including Schering-Plough's €11 billion purchase of Organon Biosciences and AstraZeneca's $15.6 billion buyout of MedImmune'(ETC 2008). Another type of pharmaco hybrid is the melding of publicly funded science with 'big pharma'; so called 'Public Private Partnerships' (PPPs). Social scientists have termed these 'co-laboratories'

(Glasner and Rothman 2004). There are a multitude of permutations in the arrangements and links between science, governance and 'big pharma', with the latter both retaining and even developing some 'in-house' research, and also outsourcing much of the R&D of (drug) product delivery. There are many different permutations of the funding and research 'co-laboratory' PPP model. For example, The Diet and Health Research Industry Club, co-funded by BBSRC, the Medical Research Council, the Engineering and Physical Sciences Research Council and 15 company members including Coca-Cola, GlaxoSmithKline and Nestlé, launched £4 million's worth of projects in 2008 'with the aim of improving scientific understanding of the key issues linking diet and health' (BBSRC 2008). One route for facilitating pharmacoG PPPs are the UK's 'Geneparks',[11] the remit of which is explained by 'Ian':

> A lot of bright ideas come out of basic research but ... the academic sectors ... have to work in partnership with commercial companies to move that into practice ... if you're making a new drug then you're going to have to have ... the investment and the time and the expertise, so you've got to work with big pharma.
>
> ('Ian')

'Ian's' role could be compared to that of a broker, facilitating deals between university labs and 'big pharma'. In contrast to the 'boom years' of DNA prospecting, 'Ian's' narrative identifies how 'big pharma' is expecting more of the early stages of R&D to be undertaken before they are prepared to take the financial risk of uptaking a project.

> if a pharmaceutical company wants to pick up that project ... if you just say ... we found the gene ... ['big pharma'] will say right, well, so what? ... come back when you know what it does. Even better, come back when you've found a drug that modulates the activity of that gene ... [or] when you've got it into pre clinical trials and you've shown its safety and its efficacy.
>
> ('Ian')

The university 'spinout company' model has been developed to translate publicly funded research into a private, potentially profit-making venture, which is likely to have links with 'big pharma' at some point in its narrative. The knowledge and other end products drift from publicly funded university science into the 'private' domain of the 'big pharma' spectrum. ETC group are amongst several NGO 'prime movers' who have researched the 'assemblages' formed by 'big pharma' in market takeovers and PPP mergers. They have been highly alert to the significance of 'big pharma' as a politically, socially and economically produced phenomenon, for example in relation to the impacts of 'market-led science' on health delivery (chapter 6), and the politics of ownership. It is increasingly difficult to identify what 'belongs' to the nation state as the output of publicly funded scientific research, and what belongs to the 'big pharma' company with a stake in the PPP, especially as the journey from lab to end product is outsourced and in-sourced in different structural formats. Patenting is a key aspect of the ownership debate (Section two).

Finally there are other sorts of pharmacoG-related 'hybrid assemblages'. In November 2003, 'Alice' was a postdoctoral researcher working as a genetic sequencer at Cambridge, UK. In discussing the production and use of genetic sequencing information, she talked about 'open source':

> I was working on structural genomics and on open source software development, EMBOSS ... European Molecular Biology Open Source Software Suite ... making genomics tools available on the internet for everybody to use, no matter who they are. And they can use them on the data that's freely available as well.
>
> ('Alice')

Alice provides a social justice rationale for 'open source'; to make software tools and accruing databases freely available to all researchers (assuming they have the hardware to use them). She said:

> People are talking about an open source pharmaceutical department ... a lot of work gets done ... in collaboration with private companies, but if that can be changed, just doing it in an open source way, then that would remove all the conflicts of interest because the companies wouldn't be involved in that field anymore ... the whole open access model has really swung a lot of opinion in biology.
>
> ('Alice')

'Alice' provides an important alternative account of routes to achieve research outcomes, very different from the innovation and competition model of economic incentive and reward which predominates in this domain. The 'open source' alternative of co-operation rather than [bio-] competition between researchers and research teams has been creating its own pathways of interactions and political spaces, perhaps in particular through the spaces opened up by UK Sanger centre and Human Genome Project initiatives. There are important historical synergies between IT, biology and open source; much of the free open source software that runs on LINUX was produced by and for biologists.[12] It is important to note that while 'Alice' combines her support for open source with an articulated, developed critique of capitalism and market forces, this is far from being a standard discourse amongst scientists working with open-source models. However there does seem to be some sense of a networked altruism:

a lot of computer people working on the genome now ... those same people could walk into jobs paying fifty, sixty, seventy grand a year. They're not; they're conscientiously going into this open source movement.

('Alice')

Being in favour of open source, however, is not necessarily a complete solution to identified concerns. First, there are still major concerns about what the information could be used for; for example, privacy and discrimination issues accruing to database use (chapter 3). Second, 'open-source' data does not preclude the information being commercially appropriated and privatised in further applications; in fact it may even facilitate this, as 'Alice' notes:

I'm sure ['big pharma'] will try and patent SNPs [Single Nucleotide Polymers] ... I think [they] are becoming aware of the fact that this is where the really interesting patents might be. And so yes, it's completely in their interests to share [genetic, genomic] data.

('Alice')

Marx wrote that all capitalist development in fact depends on the equivalent of open source or commons or sharing to start with. Others have discussed whether some of the 'open' collaborations between industry and academia can be seen as an attempt to block SMEs from enclosing valuable knowledge needed for systemic changes in the sector (Rajan 2006). Recent developments look set to shake up the field still further, with people now volunteering to make their genomes 'public' (*New Scientist* 2008b; Lunshof *et al.* 2008).

Policy and regulation

In the UK, specific regulatory frameworks and strict criteria govern the multiple fields in which pharmacoG science operates. Different pathways for drug R&D lead to multiple regulatory doors, for example ethical protocols for animal testing (Home Office 2009) and safety and ethical protocols for human clinical trial stages (Dept of Health 2004a), including informed consent criteria.[13] Pharmaco health risks such as adverse reactions to drugs are often identified in policy/legislation, for example generating strict criteria on the process of moving a drug to and through the human clinical trial stage – regulated by the Medicines and Healthcare products Regulatory Agency (MHRA).[14] The main regulatory site in the UK post approval is the National Institute for Clinical Excellence (NICE). NICE decides whether the NHS will pay for a drug,[15] and thus makes value judgements about whether it's worth paying or not. Standard risk assessments include:

1   risks in basic R&D and clinical trial stages
2   adverse reaction to drugs
3   adverse reaction to drug related bio-products

The regulatory sphere is thus another 'hybrid site', consisting of multiple bodies and institutions involved in producing and governing phamacoG. The UK government, like the EU, has given itself a mandate to exploit bio-resources and scientific knowledge to drive economic growth and this is reflected in its regulatory and policy approaches. The Department of Health has a mandate to develop the economic environment for 'big pharma' (BIS ca. 2009). Politically informed policy thus crosses into scientific practice, when EU and UK governance emphasises the importance of the pharmaco/bio-tech sector for wealth creation. In then Prime Minister Tony Blair's words: 'A successful pharmaceutical industry is a prime example of what is needed in a successful knowledge economy' (PICTF 2001).

This combination of health goals (where health is framed in terms of pharmacoG-related cures and treatments) as a 'public good', and potential economic benefits, has dominated the way in which pharmacoG is constructed in governance spheres. A narrative of a specific model of economic growth has thus emerged, linked to health priorities. From the viewpoint of global bodies that aim to promote liberal economic growth and have an interest in global health such as the Organisation for Economic Cooperation and Development (OECD),[16] this bio-economic approach should generate capital to create resources that can 'trickle-down', enabling citizens to benefit from the pharmacoG-related goods (including knowledge) and services provided at the end of the pipe. A report on an OECD pharmacogenetics conference in 2005 states that

> A number of scientific, regulatory, and economic challenges need to be overcome if pharmacogenetics is to be taken up more widely by healthcare systems ... Public policy and coordinated international action may be necessary.[17]
>
> (OECD 2009a)

EU bio-ethics committees such as the European Group on Ethics have also made statements on pharmacoG (EGE 2000) and the EU has made available a huge budget for pharmacoG related research (CEC 2007a, b).

Global 'governance' of pharmacoG exists in the form of guidelines, best practice, and the creation of institutions such as the Human Genome Organisation (HUGO) and the Human Proteome Organisation. HUGO released a pharmacoG statement emphasising the need for 'benefit sharing' (HUGO 2000). HUGO and the OECD's emphasis on 'trickle-down' and 'benefit-sharing' mechanisms show the role played by global bodies in framing ethical guidelines and principles within a Neoliberal economic framework, and again illustrate that economics, health and ethics are interrelated discourses in respect of pharmacoG. Patient and other civil society groups have influenced the debate here, around access, equity, and priorities in identifying and setting health policy. Patient-group lobbying by the Treatment Action Campaign and the influence of global players, such as the World Health Organization

(WHO), have contributed to a landmark decision whereby changes in the Trade Related Intellectual Property Rights agreement of the World Trade Organisation (WTO) changed the terms of access to drug products, through enabling copies of generic drugs to be developed, produced and sold by Third World countries (TAC 2003), catalysed by the need for people with HIV and AIDS in Africa to have access to AIDS drugs at prices that they or their health systems could afford.

International moves to identify global health priorities such as tackling AIDS, SARS and malaria have seen established bodies such as WHO and UNESCO producing reports and statements in relation to pharmacoG research (UNESCO 2003). WHO published a report identifying risks and opportunities relating to the potential translation of genetics research into global health outcomes (WHO 2002). Importantly, whilst identifying that significant medical advances would be made, this report strongly critiqued genetic hype in relation to the setting and achievement of global health priorities and goals (see chapter 8). The report was an important contribution to the debates about how health budgets should be spent.

Section two: the 'bio-economy': definitions, examples and implications

This section develops the theme of economic competitiveness and pharmacoG which has been shown to be central to much discourse from 'prime movers', including policy makers. The 'bio-economy' has been defined as 'the discourses and practices of economic competitiveness that pervade biotechnology policy-making in the UK, Europe and the USA' (Birch 2006: 2). Birch argues that it is in fact the 'future promise' discourse relating to *economic competitiveness*, as much as promissory discourse relating to *cures*, which is the major driver pushing the development of the bio-economy along a specific axis. Section One identified how health and economic development are tied together in policy frameworks accruing to pharmacoG, such as 'bio-economic' promissory discourse in EU and UK governance. Here, for example, is a quote from a EU FP7 research framework policy document, which outlines that 'FP7 is a key tool to respond to Europe's needs in terms of jobs and competitiveness, and to maintain leadership in the global knowledge economy' (CEC 2007b). Economic competitiveness is simply the way business is done; it is the default setting. A recent article on the pharmaceutical company Roche's moves into personalised pharmaco provides a standard narrative; R&D is constructed in terms of financially risky 'gambles' with high stakes; heavy losses, or huge profit (*Time* 2008).There are other shades in the bio-economic spectrum. As we have seen, the OECD invokes a concept of 'sustainable economic growth' in relation to pharmacoG product development: economic reward is seen as an incentive to innovation, with 'trickle-down' benefits.

The bio-economy is thus part of an ideological and political-economic package, generally referred to in quite generalist and loose ways (by different campaign groups, for example) such as 'globalisation', 'global capitalism', 'late capitalism', 'Neoliberal capitalism' (Tormey 2004). All accounts describe a process whereby national governance, 'big business' and international regulatory accords (such as the WTO) have aimed to further liberalise markets through a competition model which values goods, services, and resources in terms of what price they can fetch on a global money market; speculative investment, essentially. Given the spectacular collapse of the global financial system in late 2008, it is quite possible this will impact still further on this speculative market model (see chapter 8), already undergoing shocks when this interview was conducted in 2004:

> the bio tech sector has changed quite significantly over the last two or three years ... in 2001, bio tech had a very high valuation based on ... the promise of genomics ... investors have got their fingers burned.
>
> ('Ian')

UK bio-tech are now asking for direct public finance (*Telegraph* 2008). The rapidly changing nature of R&D practice within 'big pharma' over the last decade has happened as a result of lack of viable applications accruing from the genetic/genomic information – the gene sequences, and stretches of DNA – which 'big pharma' bought in the late 1990s/early 2000s and patented (*Guardian* 2000). Money was raised through the promissory discourse over the returns which investing in this resource would bring (chapter 8). Because of this, with aforementioned burned fingers, 'big pharma' is increasingly unlikely to take a chance on R&D expenditure at a basic stage, and is 'outsourcing' R&D back to universities.

Many patient groups have identified the potential for a genetic component in their disease or condition to be treated or cured with pharmacoG products. The patient group case study (chapter 1) has exceptionally strong relationships with 'big pharma' and can be seen as supportive of the bio-economic model under which 'big pharma' operates, because of the hopes for cures and treatments. 'Susan' is the spokesperson for a leading pro-research UK patient lobby group. During her interview, she discussed funding, and what she framed as the mutually beneficial relationship between her campaign group and 'big pharma':

> some of the biggest pharma companies do give us money ... Glaxo Smith Kline, Pfizer, Astra Zeneca ... we work with them because they're doing research that our members want.
>
> ('Susan')

'Susan' talked about the fact that the group had been criticised for this:

> [Critics say] 'Oh you're just funded by the drug companies' ... yes, we are and we make no bones about it ... we're working with patients and

patients don't have money. And so the people that have the money are actually quite happy that we take on the issue ... the public in general don't trust drug companies, probably don't trust scientists, but, if you're like I am, a parent of a child with a life threatening condition, they tend to trust you.

('Susan')

The patenting narrative provided later in the chapter gives a specific example of how 'Susan' and her campaign colleagues tend to support 'big pharma's' 'way of doing things'. There is perhaps a tendency amongst those critiquing 'big pharma' to forget that there are real patients behind the hype and the profit margins. 'Susan' is a prime mover, mobilising with a range of resources and across a range of networks, for very clear goals. Patient-led initiatives have had an impact on R&D and the development of applications and treatments. The scale of such mobilisation stretches from grassroots kitchen table activism, through to high-powered, extremely well resourced and well connected charities, for example the AMRC.

Promissory discourses accruing to 'pharmacoG' were of course developed in detail in Section one. The following subsections set out a number of critiques of the 'bio economy', predominantly from 'sustainability citizenship' networks.

A central discourse from policy and political frameworks is that the market is a driver of scientific and economic innovation and hence is QED 'a good thing'. Market-led science is affecting the scope, nature, direction and targets of R&D. Those prime movers (such as ETC group) critiquing the 'bio-economic' model, say that its prime concern is economic competitiveness and ensuring market share; not defining, and providing for, the health needs of populations. From their perspective, the viability of health policy deliverables and priority setting via market-led science is questionable. A short-lived European campaign network on technology and sustainability which mobilised over FP7 budget spend and the 'bio-economic' model, the European Science Social Forum Network, noted in 2005 that

Such an approach supports and judges research and innovation only in its ability to deliver moneymaking ventures, not whether it can make society a more sustainable and healthy place to live.

(ESSFN 2005)

Campaigners argue that providing economic incentives for 'big pharma' and others within the private model is simply not the best way to fund R&D or to achieve health goals. They say that the bio-economic model means that research can get funded even if it doesn't ultimately treat or cure, if the idea sounds convincing enough: 'in some senses it doesn't matter whether it 'works' or not; what's important is that finance and government are prepared to support it' ('Lucy'). The story of pharmacogenetics and associated bioscience is one of an ever-moving R&D target. The OECD notes that 'in 2007 the number of pharmacogenetics-based diagnostics on the market is still limited with less than a dozen products commercially available'.[18] There is an important issue of resource distribution here; where public (global, national) money is spent in terms of health policy, and health goals. PharmacoG is a key area of 'future promise', which campaigners argue is causing an associated lack of focus on environmental social justice routes to health goals and policy (chapter 6). Importantly, the World Health Organization has also sought to locate pharmacoG within a broader analysis of strategies for global health, citing poverty as a major cause of ill health. Thus whether the interplay of the bio-economy and pharmacoG are the best means to achieving global public health goals is contested territory. Whether it can deliver targeted applications for specific patient groups is still to be seen.

Critics argue that the 'bio-economy' is having an unhealthy impact on 'identity politics'. 'Big pharma' are very aware of the power of mobilising patient groups, and the legitimacy they have as authentic and hence trustworthy voices, articulating emotively powerful frames such as cures for sick children which resonate with 'the general public'; such discourses can mobilise important resources, sway legislatures, create allies with good political links. A recent report by Consumers International criticises drug companies for misleading consumers, and cites drug company sponsoring of patient groups funding disease awareness campaigns as a new technique in their armoury of marketing strategies (BMJ 2006, Consumers International 2006). Clever tactics employed by 'big pharma' to mimic and initiate 'genuine grassroots' patient activism have been identified, challenged, and termed 'astroturf' by activists (PR Watch 2003). There are also concerns about whether patient groups are being deliberately created as markets for products by 'big pharma'. This potential marketing of specific pharmacoG products is linked by technology watchdogs to 'syndrome invention':

> We have good evidence of [big pharma] inventing syndromes ... we have a whole literature that's been generated by the pharmaceutical companies and ... medical media [saying] ... you need to have our pills that we're offering you.
>
> ('Mike')

Consumers of a product for a newly found or described syndrome are a potential social phenomenon and very much muddy the waters about whether such bio-consumers can be called 'patients'.

On a related note, technology watchdogs such as ETC have made links with Disability Rights campaigners over 'identity politics' issues, critiquing 'geneticised' accounts of health as biologically reductive in that identity is being reduced to a set of genetic syndromes. 'Mike' notes that the 'bio-economic' model of pharmacoG is

> creating a market by re-casting people as in one way or another as defective ... a redefinition of what is healthy. And if you have an ongoing

redefinition of normal ... suddenly we will become unhealthy and with defects ... we all ... become a market for improving ourselves.

('Mike')

Campaigners see this first of all as being ethically troubling in that there are value judgements being made about what types of traits and conditions are seen as 'defective' (chapter 5). Second, there is an issue of whether market-led science simply means that products are being tailored for a market that will pay for them, and that R&D is not being focused on where there is greatest need. Further, sustainability citizenship actors critique pharmacoG as being part of a narrative of individualised responsibility for health. Campaigners argue that this may suit those who can afford to be bio-consumers of tailored products, but it further disempowers the poor. They say that those that can 'eat right for their genotype' will; those who can't will be blamed under an increasing tendency at policy level to individualise responsibility for health (*The Times* 2008b). Chapter 6 develops this important social justice critique of 'geneticisation', showing how genetic/genomic information is being used to 'blame and frame'; to place responsibility for health on the individual and discount the environmental context. Geneticised accounts can and do frame out social justice issues, such as addressing poverty and environmental causes of disease, and campaigners argue that the bio-economy encourages geneticised accounts of health to the detriment of the disadvantaged.

Section one identified the 'future promise' of personalised pharmaco, where drugs could potentially be targeted to small population sub-groups. Given the phenomenal costs of producing individualised medicine, R&D is likely to focus on the diseases of those who can afford to pay for it, if this 'future promise' manifests at all, as 'Mike' points out:

and I've seen the presentation saying; here is your market in the coming fifty years. You've got an aging population, baby boomers who are into staying young ... and they don't want to get Alzheimer's. There's a wonderful population of people who have money ... which makes sense financially, of course.

('Mike')

According to 'Mike' and others, the interests of the drug companies are in treating diseases that need long-term or lifelong treatment: hence their focus on maintaining these conditions, in finding similar conditions, and a lack of interest in conditions of the sort that tend to affect the developing world. 'Mike' identified concerns from key stakeholders that pharmacoG does little to address global health concerns: 'someone from Medicins Sans Frontières ... [spoke] about the way in which pharmaceutical companies were ... not really developing drugs that mattered to the people they [MSF] were dealing with'. Such critiques do not totally discount the potential role of pharmacoG in disease cure and prevention. Rather they contextualise the role of pharmacoG, identifying that pharmaco lobby power has the force to 'sell' its particular set of knowledge claims in the marketplace of the 'knowledge economy', drowning out other sorts of knowledge claims, such as environmental social justice.

> there are certain types of knowledge [which are] privileged with money ... that genomics brief, ... the pharmaceutical companies, that's where all the money is going. With little heading down the complementary health care route or an environmental remediation route or an epidemiological one ... there's so many other ways in which we could be approaching health, all of which are getting very little funding ... Everything is focused on the genetic route.
>
> ('Mike')

Scientific R&D is often framed per se as a public good, because it will potentially treat and cure disease. Not only is this promissory discourse questionable in terms of scientific validity, a further question is: does this mean 'anything goes'? For example, there are significant health risks accruing to research participation, such as the risks of human drugs testing (*New Scientist* 2006, Alexander 2006b). Watchdogs have voiced concerns about the framing of participation in drugs trials as an altruistic 'duty' of [bio] citizens to work towards 'public good' outcomes (Plows and Boddington 2006); see chapter 6.

Critics thus say that under market conditions, a combination of financial risk and genetic uncertainty has ensured a research focus on 'usual suspect' diseases; this is straightforwardly acknowledged by all concerned, as 'Ian' highlights:

> a lot of clinical trials fail in phase three. So ... big pharma companies are only interested in the big diseases ... cancer, cardio vascular, neurology, diabetes ... standard things. And they're not interested in something that's only got a market of ... twenty million dollars a year.
>
> ('Ian')

Similarly, campaigners argue that markets are pushing specific research directions with increased potential for biased and/or skewed results. Alice's is an important 'insider account' here:

> the whole scientific community has been stitched up by corporate interests ... people have been gagged and there's less academic freedom and independence in the biomedical area ... in America ... the pharmaceutical companies will be funding you, and you get a bias introduced into the way that you look at things.
>
> ('Alice')

GeneWatch is among several watchdogs critiquing what they believe is genomic hype from 'big pharma' in relation to profitability, pointing out that selling 'pharmacoG futures' is good for financial market share rather than for people's health (see chapters 6, 8). As set against the promissory narrative accruing to pharmacoG, the lack of products on the market perhaps speaks for itself (Nightingale and Martin 2004; Hopkins *et al.* 2007).

There are many different perspectives amongst patient groups on the role that pharmacoG might play in treating or curing their conditions. Not all patient groups support the current direction and practice of pharmaceutical research and have links with 'big pharma' and its mandate; indeed some are stridently opposed to it, and/or focus their campaigning on the environmental triggers that they think catalysed their condition (Batt 1994). These patient movements consistently frame the issues in terms of social justice and environmental issues, for example mobilising over pollution grievances (Plows and Boddington 2006; Brown and Zavestoski 2004). Importantly, locating health in a broader context of environmental and social justice is a core element of 'sustainability citizenship', and unsurprisingly there is thus significant crossover between prime movers amongst these different networks. For example, the international world health network, the People's Health Movement (PHM), is explicitly critical of 'big pharma' (PHM 2009). Health goals are focused on tackling poverty and inequity. PHM's critical analysis of the capacity of 'big pharma' and pharmacoG to contribute to global health goals, and an accompanying emphasis on equity and access issues, links it with 'sustainability citizenship' actors such as technology Watchdogs (chapter 6).

Thus although certain patient and other groups critique pharmaco *profits*, they do not necessarily reject the *products* – the drugs – pharmaco may potentially provide. Most of the specific critiques of 'big pharma' from patients and others relate to issues of access and equity: problems stem from ... unequal access to health services and medications and treatments ... the pharmaceutical companies are a target for anti globalisation [action] ... about access' ('Alice'). Patient groups mobilising for better treatments and cures can critique power relations blocking their access to drugs, and even mobilise in confrontational ways in relation to pharmaco, even when they still need the specific pharmaco product. In Seoul in February 2003 activists occupied Novartis head office in order to protest about the high cost of the anti-sarcoma drug Glivec.[19] They opposed the company rather than supported it, even though they needed the product. AIDS patients are the usually quoted example (Bucchi 2004; Rose and Novas 2004) of vocal, internationally mobilising networks, which have taken up issues of access and distributory justice.

A key frame for watchdogs such as ETC and GeneWatch relates to the commodification and ownership of bio-resources and the patenting of bio-information; this is an ethical and political analysis based on the idea of the patenting of bio-information as 'New Enclosures', and an accompanying critique of the profit-making function of 'big pharma' which plunders these resources. Lobbying and awareness raising about access and equity by groups has contributed to the uptake of 'benefit-sharing' mechanisms by global governance such as HUGO. Regulatory bodies tend to focus on mitigating some of the damage caused by patenting within an existing Neoliberal framework (through benefit sharing, for instance) rather than preventing the damage in the first place or exploring other research practices and goals; while a campaign group like ETC frames its critiques through a critical account of capitalism.

Patents are an important example of 'the bio-economy' in action and a well established site of public contention, not to mention ambivalence. Patents are part of a suite of internationally recognised Intellectual Property tools which are awarded for original inventions to reward the 'inventor' and provide incentives for research. But what counts as an invention, especially in relation to biological and living organisms or parts thereof? Although patents were designed largely for mechanical inventions, in the last 20 years they have been awarded for 'everything under the sun' (Diamond v Chakrabarty 1980), including DNA sequences; specific genes; proteomic sequences; Single Nucleotide Polymorphisms (SNPs); technological applications such as mass spectrometry machines; stem cell lines; bio-engineered tissue, and cloned animals (OncoMouse^{TM} – Haraway 1991). Multilateral and international patent agreements always existed, policed through the World Intellectual Property Organization (WIPO). A strategy to get patents into a trade agreement involves the WTO.

> The WTO only sets minimum standards for member countries' intellectual property laws and does not get involved in individual patents ... that is up to each country to handle according to its own laws and its own approaches (and these can vary considerably) ... several governments have signed agreements with each other cooperating on patent registration, and WIPO does have facilities to help patent applicants seek protection for their inventions around the world, for a fee.
>
> (WTO spokesperson in personal email, June 2003)

National law is thus highly important, even within Europe and the EU. Different countries within the EU and internationally have different patent laws, meaning the entire field is increasingly the subject of lengthy court battles over who has ownership (OCA 2003), and what counts as innovation. Within the UK, the Intellectual Property Office sets standards, and these have shifted over time in relation to what is seen as a legitimate 'invention'. Reflecting changes in the way bioinfomatics has changed the innovation landscape in relation to 'mapping' genetic and genomic sequences, patents are no longer routinely awarded to sequenced stretches of DNA (IPO 2009).

As part of a broader bio economic governance framework, patents have thus been located as a key incentive to innovation and research, with 'trickle-down' benefits. While this remains the 'dominant paradigm' position, there are cracks running through this construction. Watchdogs such as ETC say that patenting genetic/genomic information and bio-resources, is the enclosure of 'public goods' and oppose it per se. ETC defines such patenting as 'bio-piracy' and emphasises the inequalities surrounding the appropriation of bio-resources: 'Intellectual property has become a powerful tool to enhance corporate monopoly and consolidate market power ... The ETC group opposes exclusive monopoly control over living organisms and biological processes' (ETC 2009). Such debates about 'privatising life', 'privatising nature' were prevalent during the UK GM crops campaigns of the late 1990s and are also currently invoked in relation to nanobiotechnology (Plows and Reinsborough 2008). Environmental and 'anti globalisation' activists and NGOs in the late 1990s were highly vocal in linking concerns about globalisation with specific instances of the privatisation of global 'public goods' (Purdue 2000; Plows 2004), the appropriation of resources by global elites, and the accruing social fallout in terms of equity and access. The oft-cited example in relation to human genetics is the patent of the BRCA1 and 2 genes by the company Myriad genetics (WIPO 2006). As a form of 'single gene disorder', these specific genes have been identified as 80 per cent likely to predispose to a specific form of breast cancer. Myriad genetics ownership of the BRCA 1 and 2 patents compels users to pay Myriad for the BRCA 1/2 screening even if not provided by Myriad itself.

The Indigenous Peoples Council (Harry *et al.* 2000; Howard 2001) have long been alert to the 'mining' of their DNA as a resource, and have lobbied around issues of power, ownership and the profits accruing to resulting patents. The line in the sand position, which is opposed to patenting of DNA, genes and bio-material per se, blurs when groups can simultaneously argue along more reformist lines, for benefit sharing (discussed in chapter 3) accruing to the profits made from any applications (drugs) of their genetic information.

Patents produce a range of ambivalent responses amongst patient groups, scientists and industry players. The patient case study is proactively 'pro patent':

> we went to Strasbourg, to the European Parliament ... in 1997, and we lobbied on behalf of the bio patenting directive ... we were fighting the Greens ... It was 'patents for people' basically ... our funders – ['big pharma'] wanted to patent certain technologies ... and use the money they got from that to fund research on the less popular conditions. So we were backing that and also we were backing it because if it hadn't happened, a lot of our science was going to move abroad.
>
> ('Susan')

'Susan's' account of patents as an economic incentive mirrors that of the scientific entrepreneurs and governance frameworks keen to promote the UK as a sound site for investment, research and development. Other patient groups have taken a different approach. The PXE case (PXE 2004) involved a 'prime mover' patient group opposed to patenting because they believe it blocks research. But the group took out a patent themselves on the PXE gene, so as to give the genetic information free to research teams. Flagging aforementioned concerns about benefit-sharing, 'Peter' noted that 'the charity commission ... does expect charities ... to take out patents but ... to then make the licence to technology in the public interest. Cancer Research UK has just ... pledged two licences completely for free ... for the NHS' ('Peter'). The UK's Royal Society (Britain's leading science establishment lobby, consisting of the most eminent scientists, engineers and technologists from the UK and the Commonwealth) has also made strong statements criticising the patenting process (Royal Society 2003). These criticisms primarily stem from the premise that patenting holds back research by hindering the flow of information around the 'scientific community'. The Royal Society does not focus on the access and equity issues central to ETC's critiques of bio-patenting, still less critique the dominant market model of the 'bio-economy' or the role of 'big pharma' per se. However, the Royal Society's opposition to patenting does critique the efficacy of this specific market mechanism as a means of providing health outcomes, and this represents a significant area of crossover with 'watchdog' campaign groups. Even 'big pharma' is becoming disenchanted with patents, because legal battles over patents are dragging out research timescales and costs: 'even some of the companies now are questioning whether it was really a good idea. And that's largely because the lawyers are getting all the money, nobody knows who owns what'('Peter').

Conclusion

The narrative provided in this chapter has enabled an understanding of 'pharmacoG' as hybrid field, in the process identifying some of the broader debates on pharmacoG beyond discourses of disease cure, including emergent socio-political, economic and ethical concerns. Not least among these public concerns is that the dominance of pharmacoG product-driven philosophy has swept the direction of genomic medicine away from other possibilities such as understanding environmental processes in relation to genetics, to make for better epidemiological interventions (including proactive health practices that reduce the need for medical intervention or treatment). These accounts of disease prevention from 'sustainability citizenship' actors do not exclude the role of pharmacoG in identifying and treating specific types of disease but they are extremely critical of 'bio-hype' in promissory, 'geneticised' accounts of cures (chapters 6, 8). Issues of ownership, intellectual property and access are also key frames for these prime movers and others.

In describing what 'pharmacoG' *is*, this chapter has discussed some of the processes, products and promises that pharmacoG provides and some of the key risk and benefit frames accruing to these. Much promissory discourse about 'personalised pharmaco' relates to the identification of tiny variations in genetic, genomic and proteomic expression within an individual. The promise of these products is a source of great hope for many patient groups, their advocates and members of 'disease communities'. However according to some publics, there are reasons to be critical about how the products (or the idea of them) and specifically targeted potential consumers of these products, are part of the driving economic force that are shaping this hybrid medical science/industry area, and the implications for public health goals. The chapter has provided narratives of concern around the targeting of specific publics as consumers of potential bio-products. The engagement, not to mention the construction, of publics as patients and as consumers are themes developed further in chapter 5 which, as part of a broader narrative of genetic testing and screening, further discusses issues of identity, responsibility and related ethical concerns accruing to the commercial sale of genetic/genomic tests that have been a core output of pharmacoG-related research.

5   Genetic testing and screening

Introduction

Genetic information is increasingly acknowledged to play an important role in disease expression (chapters 3, 4). The capacity to test individuals for genetic disorders is also increasing. There is diagnostic testing to confirm the presence of a condition; pre-symptomatic testing for individuals who may be at risk of developing a condition; prenatal testing to identify the presence of a condition before birth; pre-implantation testing of embryos produced through IVF; and population screening, where members of specific populations susceptible to particular conditions are tested.

This chapter highlights the complex relationship between genetic information and disease knowledge, and how different publics are negotiating this terrain. Chapter 4 identified that there have been rapid developments in sequencing and identification of SNP gene 'markers', meaning there is more raw genetic data (which may, or may not, translate into accurate genetic *knowledge* about what this data *means*). The range of available genetic tests in multiple contexts, from prenatal to adult testing, is rapidly widening. The increase of genetic testing within public healthcare, and in the spread of commercially available genetic/genomic test kits (Wallace 2008b; GeneWatch 2007; Lunshof *et al.* 2008; Prainsack *et al.* 2008) make this one of the most important arenas of public engagement with human genetics, where many debates about the meanings and implications of genetic information are being situated. The chapter shows that these tests raise complex ethical minefields which must be negotiated. Some see this as the (eugenic) 'slippery slope'; others frame tests in relation to a right to choose on the basis of new information. For many, genetic testing and screening informs debates on health and identity, human value and human nature, and social justice and equity. The accuracy of the tests, especially in relation to the predictability of multifactorial disease and assessing predisposition and at-risk status, is also a heavily contested arena.

Section one provides an overview of genetic screening and testing practice and policy, using evidence of single-gene disorders. Using examples of the prime movers who are engaging with the debates, Section two focuses on two examples of genetic testing; prenatal testing and commercially available adult testing, both of which were catalysing significant public engagement during the research timeframe. This section addresses some of the emergent issues and the ways in which they are being framed by different publics, such as issues of choice, value and 'slippery slopes' in relation to prenatal testing; while commercially available genetic tests raise issues such as how consumers will negotiate risk and what it is they are being sold. The issue of commercially driven patient/consumer identities, discussed in chapter 4, is returned to here.

Section one: a testing and screening narrative

Genetic 'screening' is a term used where genetic (or other) tests are performed on large sections or sub-sections of the population. An example is cervical cancer screening (NHS 2004). Genetic 'testing' is generally used in the context of tests targeted at individuals or families known as, or suspected of, being at increased risk of certain types of genetic disease. Chadwick *et al.* state that

> 'Genetic screening' is defined by the Danish Council of Ethics (1993) as the study of the occurrence of a specific gene or chromosome complement in a population or population group. The Council of Europe in its 'Statement on Genetic Testing' (1992) adds that there should be no previous suspicion that any given individual has the condition; the Nuffield Council on Bioethics (1993) that there should be no evidence that any given individual does, thus replacing a subjective test with an objective one. Thus although in some literature 'screening' and 'testing' are not clearly distinguished and while there are some common issues, genetic screening is defined differently than genetic testing. 'Testing' applies to individuals for whom there is some reason to think they may be 'at risk', e.g., because of family history.
>
> (Chadwick *et al.* 1998: 257)

Important differences therefore exist between genetic screening being offered as part of 'standard' population-wide healthcare (e.g. the prenatal test for Down's syndrome) – the 'opt out' approach – and genetic tests as 'opt in' for specific individuals, families or 'disease communities'.

There are thousands of multifactorial conditions with a genetic component which interacts with environmental factors. There are also over 10,000 human diseases caused by defects in single genes (Primrose and Twyman 2006); the majority of these are extremely rare.[1] Far more common, however, are the so–called 'single-gene disorders' BRCA1 breast cancer, Cystic Fibrosis (CF), Duchenne's Muscular Dystrophy, haemochromatosis, haemophilia and Huntington's disease. While these conditions share single-gene provenance, it should not render them alike in many other ways. Single-gene disorders differ in transmission patterns,[2] penetrance, available interventions and treatments, morbidity and familial scope. For example:

- Huntington's disease is an autosomal dominant disorder with complete penetrance; any person inheriting the gene will develop the condition. It is an incurable, fatal neurodegenerative disease with onset usually in mid-life. The condition involves the severe and progressive loss of nerve cells in the brain. This results in gradually increasing dementia and eventually requires full nursing care.
- Cystic Fibrosis (CF) is an incurable condition and causes breathing difficulties, chronic respiratory infections and ongoing problems with digestion. It is a recessive disease; copies of the defective gene need to be inherited from both parents.
- Haemochromatosis is a treatable recessive genetic disorder where high levels of iron are absorbed in the gut, causing excessive iron storage in organs such as the liver. Without identification and treatment serious conditions including diabetes and arthritis develop in middle age.
- Duchenne's muscular dystrophy (DMD) is a fatal X-linked condition and much more common in males than females. It is a severe muscle-wasting disorder which presents in infancy leading to most affected individuals becoming wheelchair-dependent before adolescence.
- Haemophilia is a treatable recessive X-linked condition caused by malfunctioning genes on the X chromosome and again more common in males than females. In recent years the condition has been treated successfully with the regular injection of purified blood-clotting agents.
- Some single-gene conditions may have also incomplete penetrance; that is, only some individuals with inherited mutations will be susceptible to expressing a condition. For example, not all people with a mutation in the BRCA1 gene will develop breast cancer. Potentially susceptible individuals can also choose prophylactic interventions such as surgery.

The differing forms of intervention, the age of onset and the severity of symptoms mean that single-gene disorders differ more than the simple description of genetic provenance suggests. Indeed, whilst the early focus has been on describing disease expression, the additional identification of susceptibility to a condition (e.g. BRCA1) also raises important issues regarding carrier status. A carrier of a genetic mutation will not manifest the condition[3] but could, if she or he reproduces with another carrier, produce offspring that express the disease.

Genetic information can bring with it important disease-expressive knowledge, knowledge that impacts family members and on future reproductive decision-making. Moreover, any decision to generate genetic information is replete with social, ethical and legal consequences.

What to test? When to test? Who to test?

Genetic testing refers to testing an individual, albeit with potentially family-associated consequences. However, it is also possible to screen populations rather than test individuals. Members of a defined population, who do not necessarily perceive they are at risk of – or are already affected by – a disease or its complications, are asked a question or offered a test to identify those individuals who are more likely to be helped than harmed by further tests or treatment to reduce the risk of a disease or its complications (HGC and UKNSC 2005). A very important development has been the contested introduction of prenatal tests for Down's syndrome (NICE 2008; Buckley and Buckley 2008). Moreover, the introduction of newborn screening programmes (e.g. thalassemia screening in the United Kingdom) also has to deal with the ethical implications of identifying all newborn carriers.

There is much debate regarding which conditions should be tested for, and whether tests should be expanded in population screening programmes. For example, the appropriateness of genetically testing children is conventionally seen as problematic, especially in circumstances where there is no immediate medical benefit to the child such as testing for carrier status and for adult onset disorders. There are competing ethical principles of autonomy, beneficence (the aim to produce benefit) and non-maleficence (the aim to avoid harm) at stake (Hogben and Boddington 2005). Gibson noted that: 'The attack on disease must not be meddlesome; the desire to do something must be guided by sure argument that good will come of it' (Gibson 1933). Boddington and Gregory (2008) discuss the value of information in relation to individual competence and consent. Section Two highlights how specific interest groups, such as patient groups, automatically frame information in terms of a 'right to choose', implying a capacity to negotiate information.

It has also been suggested that tests that identify conditions for which no cure or treatment exists are more 'exceptional' (chapter 6) than those that detect conditions that can be treated or prevented (SACGT 2001; HGC 2002). For example, the genetic test for Huntington's disease, which identifies individuals who will almost certainly develop an incurable, fatal neurodegenerative disease in mid-life, is considered exceptional. On the contrary, the genetic test for phenylketonuria (PKU), which identifies a condition that can be effectively treated in newborns but, if undetected, can cause serious harm, is not considered exceptional but is routinely performed in the UK (Saukko *et al.* 2006). McConkie-Rosell and DeVellis (2000) have argued that in X-linked disorders there is a possibility of a real threat of a diminished self-concept where carrier status is discovered.

A range of genetic tests are available at prenatal, post natal, child and adult levels. Prenatal tests on the embryo are carried out via two procedures. Prenatal Genetic Diagnosis (PND) 'is a type of test which is person and condition specific and aims to provide a diagnosis of the particular genetic condition the baby might have' (HGC 2004). This is amniocentesis or chorionic villus sampling, carried out on a foetus in the mother's womb complemented with maternal blood tests and ultrasound. Amniocentesis tests of the embryo carries risks of miscarriage. PreImplantation Genetic Diagnosis (PGD) is a technique where embryos created outside the body by IVF can be tested to see if they have a genetic disorder. One or two cells are removed for testing from the embryo at the 6–10 cell stage ... Implantation into the woman's uterus will generally only be attempted for embryos without the genetic disorder.

(HGC 2004)

Testing was for a specific disorder prior to 2009, when a new 'karyomapping' technique was developed that can test embryos for almost any inherited disease (*The Times* 2009); this has yet to become standard policy practice and is likely to generate debate.

PND and PGD are used to identify traits and in specific circumstances, to 'select out' embryos carrying these traits, or to select embryos with specific traits ('saviour siblings'). Examples of conditions for which both kinds of prenatal test (PND and PGD) are used include Down's syndrome; a specific form of congenital deafness (this exists as a population screening programme in Italy (Coviello *et al.* 2004)); Duchenne's muscular dystrophy; cystic fibrosis; cleft palate; Tay Sachs; and susceptibility tests for specific types of cancer known to have a strong genetic component, including specific forms of bowel and breast (BRCA1 and 2) cancer. There is also the option of sex selection for 'medical' purposes, for X-linked diseases such as Duchennes and Haemophilia.

PGD is also now able to be used (on a case by case basis) to create 'saviour siblings'; the IVF implantation of a foetus following PGD, where the implanted foetus is identified as a genetic match for a sibling. The 'saviour sibling' might be able to provide stem cells from the birth cord for the 'sick sibling'. The potential to test for, and select, the sex of a foetus via PGD raised the issue of sex selection for 'non-medical', 'family balancing' reasons. The Masterton case (Wilkinson 2008) catalysed emotive debates on this issue.

Tests on newborns and children are also carried out. On newborns, the standard test is a heel prick for a blood sample, to identify specific traits/ conditions; generally, to establish the presence of a specific, heritable, 'serious' disorder such as CF. The Dept of Health (2003) flagged the possibility of a newborn genetic screening policy (referred to by some as a 'baby barcode'). Childhood testing takes DNA samples from blood, saliva and skin, again to identify specific traits, usually to establish the presence of a specific, heritable, 'serious' disorder such as CF, or in certain cases a late onset disorder; or also to determine carrier status.

Adult testing follows a similar pattern. Tests are taken using range of bio-samples, most often blood, saliva, skin, semen. Tests are commercially available as well as being offered to patients within the NHS, and are undertaken for a range of reasons. The most common are to identify adult-onset disease, to confirm familial inheritance patterns, to identify carrier status, for 'non-medical' purposes (for example, paternity). Generally within the NHS, adult testing is for 'serious' 'single-gene' disorders such as early onset Alzheimer's, Parkinson's and Huntington's disease.

Policy and regulation

The vast spectrum of tests and screens, from prenatal to adult, and the variety of end goals, means that there are a wide range of different regulatory and policy bodies and frameworks, and associated advisory groups and committees. This section provides a very broad overview of some key legislative and policy players, with some specific examples of issues which are the subject of policy and ethical debate.

A key policy actor is National Screening Committee (NSC), which 'assesses proposed new screening programmes against a set of internationally recognised criteria covering the condition, the test, the treatment options and effectiveness and acceptability of the screening programme' (NSC 2005). The HFEA covers embryonic legislation (prenatal testing and screening), with the 2008 Act (Dept of Health 2008c) (see chapter 2) setting a broad umbrella remit, and sex selection for 'family balancing' reasons is a key area where a line has been clearly drawn. Current UK policy is that all women be offered the first trimester combined test for Down's syndrome (NICE 2008). Adult and childhood testing and policy represents a vast area of legislation, a few examples of which include the current moratorium on the use of genetic information for insurance purposes agreed between the Department of Health and Association of British Insurers in 2005 (Dept of Health and ABI 2005). Here 'Angela' discusses the regulatory moratorium in the context of its status as a public 'hot topic' in 2004:

> One of the biggest topics is genetics and insurance ... any public meetings we have around that are always pretty much over subscribed. A lot of interest but also a lot of concern because of the potential for using adverse test results, and I think that it brought a possible mistrust of how the industry actually works. That's ... a 'sexy' topic.
>
> ('Angela')

European regulatory links with the UK were discussed by 'Angela':

> 'we need to keep an eye out on what's happening with the European Union, to bring those directives and the potential impact that might have on areas of interest both to Commissions first and to the Department of Health more broadly'

Advisory bodies work closely with those making policy, in particular the Human Genetics Commission (HGC) and NCoB, producing a number of reports. A joint HGC and NSC report was called *Profiling the Newborn*[4] (HGC and NSC 2005). The HGC also ran the *Choosing the future* public consultation document on PND and PGD (HGC 2004). The UK Genetic Testing Network is an example of a (by now familiar) hybrid model of governance, which 'advises the NHS on genetic testing [and] brings together all the people involved in providing genetic tests for inherited disorders' (UKGTN

2008). The network includes clinical genetics counsellors, scientists involved in test development, and the patient group Genetic Interest Group (GIG).

'Ian' further highlights the hybridity of 'the science' as research site, as potential application, and policy/governance:

> We have interactions with the NHS ... through health services research ... if you have a new diagnostic test it becomes part of something called the UK genetic testing network. So there's a whole series of. ... justifications, applications ... to get this onto the portfolio ... So we obviously have to work with those guys very closely.
>
> ('Ian')

Regulation and bio-ethical codes of practice around 'informed consent' and genetic counselling practice has been developed in relation to familial testing and heritability, most notably in the context of 'single gene' conditions where having the gene means a specific condition will be expressed. In relation to familial traits and genetic testing, therefore, protocols, policy, bio-ethics principles (to test or not to test, informed consent protocols for children and adults) are relatively well established (Clarke 1998). Information generated through genetic testing is frequently articulated in policy discourse, in degrees of seriousness, and it seems that relative significance or severity is also presented differentially to produce the differing recommendations with respect to carrier and predictive testing (Boddington and Hogben 2006a, 2006b). These issues have been discussed with especial attention being paid to the value of childhood genetic testing (see Borry *et al.* 2006, 2008; Hogben and Boddington 2005) which raises specific issues about consent, the benefits to the child. There have been recent calls for testing to be allowed under 16; when the child reaches 'reproductive age' (Borry *et al.* 2006). This is supported with arguments explaining that under-16-year-olds (the age of sexual consent in the UK) are generally entitled to seek and receive medical care for contraception and pregnancy (Clayton 2008).

There has in recent years been a debate within the philosophical literature, with implications for policy, on the right to know and the right not to know genetic information. Because genetic information about one person may be revealed automatically by revealing information about relatives, or as the result of other tests such as paternity tests, it is sometimes necessary for some individuals to argue specifically for the right *not* to know. In relation to adult testing specifically, very often, when a patient has or carries a genetic condition, there will be other family members who might benefit from knowing that they too are at risk of this condition. For example, there might be surveillance treatment or prophylaxis that could be offered, or the knowledge might be relevant to reproductive decision-making. Is the patient then obligated in any way to pass on this information? And, if the patient refuses to do so, should medical staff be at liberty to divulge the information?

Because of such issues, there are regular suggestions that rules of confidentiality and privacy of knowledge should be amended to recognise that genetic information does not just 'belong' to the individual patient, but to the family as a whole (Skene 2001). Resistance to this idea is strong as it breaks a central pillar of medical ethics, the confidentiality belonging to the patient–doctor relationship (Ngwena and Chadwick 1993). For example, in relation to Huntington's disease, despite the possibility of testing, many at-risk individuals have declined, and take-up remains low. For various reasons, many prefer to exercise their right 'not to know'. Many have children without ascertaining their carrier status. This can cause difficulties. For example, if the adult child of an at-risk individual has the test, and it proves positive, this means that their at-risk parent certainly also has the gene. This may be knowledge they did not want to have (Parker and Lucassen 2003). This issue represents an emergent legal and policy tangle.

As with stem cell regulation (chapter 2), the UK combines a large amount of regulation with a liberal policy practice, with some significant precedent setting. In terms of policy standard setting, critics argue that there is a tendency for a 'one size fits all' case basis for policy where a 'single gene', 'severe condition' example stands in for other conditions, where there is less of a genetic component or where the implications of having the gene are less 'severe'. A compelling 'single case' example, such as the HFEA 'saviour siblings' ruling (HFEA 2001), can set a benchmark on what could be seen as a 'slippery slope', subsequently codified by the Human Fertilisation and Embryology Act 2008 (Dept of Health 2008c) which authorised an even broader remit, including regulating the creation of human embryos outside the body. Similarly, it is important to be careful in generalising from one genetic disease to another. Huntington's disease is considered a very serious neurological disease, which attacks at variable age but generally in the prime of life; it is seen as highly burdensome, is untreatable and fatal. For these reasons, a degree of reluctance to test for this condition may or may not have implications for other adult-onset disorders. It is noteworthy that this condition is frequently referred to in ethical and policy discussion papers.

Finally, there is very little, or no, actual regulation in relation to commercially available adult tests for a range of 'genetic conditions', large numbers of which are increasingly available online. The Nuffield Council on Bioethics published a report (NCoB 2002) recommending 'kite-marks' guaranteeing a standard for adult genetic tests, noting that the combination of the internet and the free market was making national regulation of individual consumer behaviour almost impossible.

Section two: prenatal testing and commercial adult testing: key issue frames

Prenatal genetic testing

Section one provided an overview of what prenatal tests consist of and why they are carried out; to screen out traits, or on occasion to select for traits ('saviour siblings'). 'Saviour siblings' were a key focus of public debate in relation to PGD during the research timeframe. A 'saviour sibling' is created following IVF implantation of a specific embryo after PGD; the implanted embryo is a genetic match for an existing sibling suffering a serious, generally terminal, genetic condition. The hope is that the IVF baby – the 'saviour sibling' – will be able to donate bio-material, generally from the birth cord, which would be a genetic match for the ill child, potentially leading to a cure.[5] 'Saviour siblings' catalysed significant engagement by 'the general public' for example in the UK in July 2004 around a specific Human Fertilisation and Embryology Authority (HFEA) policy precedent-setting case (PET 2004). There was much discussion of 'designer babies' in relation to this case; not 'designer babies' in the sense of engineered reproductive clones, the stuff of science fiction, but from the capacity to choose, even in a limited way, the genetic characteristics of a baby via IVF. An online BBC thread in 2004 framed the issue in these terms: 'The fertility watchdog has decided to relax the rules over the creation of so-called 'designer babies'. (BBC 2004b). Much of the 2004 public debate on this chat thread and in other public media forums such as a BBC Radio 4 phone-in programme in late 2003[6] focused on 'where to draw the line'; 'saviour siblings' signalling a 'boundary object' of public acceptability, even for potential cures for a child with a fatal condition. Many framed the issue in terms of the 'slippery slope', and were uncomfortable with the case by case policy approach. 'Playing God' was also a frame used by some members of the public. Others countered that anything which could potentially save the life of a terminally ill child was worth it. A related counter-argument is that people have babies for all sorts of reasons, and that to conceive a 'saviour sibling' is no different, invoking the genetic exceptionalism debate (chapter 6). Another recurring public concern was whether saviour siblings represented the commodification of the child, the child-as-product. These concerns have been raised repeatedly by the watchdog Human Genetics Alert (HGA 2003).[7] Importantly, while the public debates were often framed initially in quite polarising ways by different media formats, the range and depth of public responses showed quite clearly that publics were confident in negotiating highly ambivalent and complex terrain.

Some of the key debates which prenatal testing has catalysed, and the ways in which these issues have been framed, are summarised in the following subsections, followed by examples of some of the issues raised by different publics in relation to commercial adult testing.

Choice, a major focus in chapter 7, is an important frame in relation to prenatal testing and screening – PGD and PND – where these are specifically reproductive choices, a term with an important feminist legacy.

> in the ... [HGC] consultation document on reproductive decision making ... some people think screening is all about eugenics, so you ...

have to take that on board and address those sorts of concerns, and balance it out with other issues like informed choice.

('Angela')

The 'informed choice' debate is an important one, especially when couched in broad terms of understanding what it is which is being 'chosen' – and who has the right to choose, and where these 'choices' are coming from – and who is deciding that we should make them. How are people being informed and by whom? Prenatal genetic testing and screening catalyses and synthesises a range of contested and varying versions of informed choice, individual choice and informed consent. For example, Libertarianism, and different positions within feminism, will point either to a prioritising of individual autonomy in relation to 'the right to choose', or instead to how social structure, culture and power relations underlies these 'individual choices'.

The broadly 'pro genetics' patient groups (chapter 1; SIMR, AMRC, GIG) and other groups to which they are allied such as the Institute of Ideas and Progress Educational Trust are, generally speaking, in favour of the availability of genetic tests, both for identifying adult-onset conditions and also for what is generally framed as reproductive decision-making ('informed choice') in relation to prenatal screening and testing. Genetic testing is tied up with 'future promise' (chapter 8) discourses accruing to health and security; the predictability, and management, of conditions. The wish to avoid unnecessary pain and suffering are constant 'givens' in the debate on prenatal screening for 'serious' conditions. 'Knowledge is power' discourse is also common; specific patient group campaigners say that they want access to the information in order to make life choices, be better informed, be able to pass this information on to family members, and so forth; for example, to make life decisions about reproduction if one has, or carries, a gene which codes for a specific disease or trait. For example, 'Susan' said 'now "Emily" [her daughter, born with CF] luckily can find out if a child she ever has will have CF ... and it's her right to have it and it's nobody's right to stop her having it, that's the way round I see it'. Prenatal testing at the request of the family for a heritable 'serious' disease such as CF is something which the majority of interviewees were often supportive of, or at the very least sympathetic to:

> Screening for a genetic disease that is in the parent's family, these parents don't want to have another child with this disease ... Which is fair enough ... And cystic fibrosis ... If I've got one kid with that I really don't want another ... because there's so much pain in that child's life.

('Alice')

However in relation to prenatal/embryonic testing for CF specifically, the fact that these are ambivalent and complex issues is also very clear. Here is 'Peter' talking about debates about CF within a charity:

for a long time they were kind of okay [with CF] testing ... for carrier status and then you have various options ... you can just go ahead and try and have a selective abortion, or you could do PGD ... but they've moved away from that because what they're saying now is that for the Cystic Fibrosis children who are born now, as long as they are detected earlier and treated properly then you've got quite a hopeful life expectancy, and therefore we don't feel it's appropriate anymore to kind of get rid of these people, that's not the way we want to do it, and they've had I think a fairly sophisticated debate within the charity about that and this is their policy now.

('Peter')

These are not easy issues to navigate, and the majority of patients framing discourses of informed choice in relation to their support for genetic tests also identify how difficult these choices are, particularly in relation to PGD. This even more contested territory when there are PGD tests which identify 'predisposition to' (e.g. BRCA1 and 2) i.e. where it is not clear whether the disease will in fact express itself, or when, but the identified gene 'strongly predisposes' to this outcome. Other perspectives such as 'Alice's, locate the individual choice in a social context.

It's very hard territory because the Mum doesn't actually have the choice because you know, if she chooses to have her baby say with Down's syndrome ... they're quite happy kids ... She's going to be discriminated against then, [so] the choice has been made for her ... She can't afford to have a child like that. She can only afford to have an acceptably normal child.

('Alice')

Chapter 7 returns to feminist debates around the sphere of reproduction and the body and the discourse of 'choice' in relation to testing. Some feminists have felt uneasy about what they see as the misappropriation of discourse on 'the right to choose' to mean 'anything goes'. There is an interesting flip side to the discourse of choice; namely individualised responsibility, which can be linked by powerful others (e.g. governance) to debates on [bio] citizenship (chapter 6). Rights can also enrol responsibilities: to 'do the right thing'. This felt sense of responsibility may affect women's reproductive choices. In the context of prenatal screening and screening of embryos especially, certain patient group prime movers and their allies argue strongly in favour of 'the right to choose'. Framing the issues accruing to prenatal testing around the 'right to informed choice' can imply – wrongly – that to voice any concern or opposition to prenatal testing and screening means one is 'anti choice', as 'Sally' identifies:

[reproductive choice is] used as a stick against [Disability Rights (DR) groups] when we challenge prenatal testing, and this is one of the reasons why we've not seen any real direct campaigning on it in our movement, because people are frightened by this prospect that we could be seen as anti-feminist.

('Sally')

A 'slippery slope' is a progression from one position, deemed acceptable, through a series of small, possibly imperceptible changes, until we arrive at another position, deemed unacceptable. It is a commonly heard public discourse in relation to prenatal testing and screening: '[we] keep moving down that sliding slope ... what's [defined as] normal just keeps moving' ('Mike'); 'we should be careful about [having] a step by step approach ... careful about not going down a slippery slope.' (John Sulston)[8]

'Drawing lines' is another related frame: 'Where do you draw the line between wanting a baby genetically matched so as to save the life of a sibling and wanting to distinguish between a perfect and slightly imperfect foetus?' (BBC 2004); 'How and where do we draw the lines?' (ISESCO 2005). One response to such slopes is to find a way to stop them: to draw a line where clear demarcation can be made so that the slide down the slope does not go 'too far'. This might be a matter of degree. An example of this might be to say that prenatal diagnosis and selective abortion might be allowed for 'serious' conditions only. This will stop the slide towards allowing selective abortion for minor or treatable conditions such as myopia. Or it might be a matter of kind, for example that selective abortion is permissible only for monogenetic diseases; or for medical conditions but not for enhancement. One response is to say that we should not get onto the slope in the first place, as there will be no way of stopping the slide. Scepticism might be expressed that there could be any clear demarcation, for instance that disagreement about what counts as a 'serious' condition will arise, or that ideas about seriousness will change over time; this concern comes up repeatedly in research data. For example cleft palate, once held as an example of a condition that would not be screened out, now often is. This is an argument not to allow any selective termination. A response to this might be that only families with experience of such problems can judge the matter, that a 'liberal eugenics' allows parents to make these decisions for their offspring. However, accounts of liberal eugenics generally keep a role for society at large to delineate for what range of conditions is prenatal testing and screening an option.

A key issue for 'sustainability citizenship' (chapter 1) prime movers is power; not only where one individually might draw the line, but 'who is drawing it, who has the power and who will enforce it?' ('Lucy'). 'We know from experience ... it's this slippery slope, they're starting with these few things but later there'll be a lot more things and who is going to get to decide where that line is drawn' ('Sally'). Generally, policymakers decide 'where to draw the line': 'one of the issues is, pretty much where do we set limits, where do we draw the line and that's also with respect to PGD but also more broadly with respect to screening because this actually affects a lot more people' ('Angela'). Slippery slope arguments are routinely pooh-poohed, as if they are simple scaremongering to a bleak dystopian future. A slippery slope in attitudes to, and practice concerning, abortion in relation to trait de-selection has in fact occurred. Once the concept of testing for/screening out has occurred in principle, one is on the 'slippery slope' and the debate moves to where lines are drawn.

Drawing a very clear line in relation to prenatal screening/testing are the religious/faith and pro-life groups, such as Comment on Reproductive Ethics (CORE). Pro-life and religious perspectives on the embryo were discussed in chapter 2. These groups tend to have 'embryo-centric' framings of the PGD and PND debate, and the status of the embryo has been a highly visible black and white discourse in the public sphere in relation to prenatal genetic testing. In chapter 2 and also in this chapter, the 'volume has been turned down' on line-drawing over the status of the embryo, with less attention paid to these actors in comparison to the case study groups and networks. The rationale for so doing is that this is an overly reified trope which has dominated the framing of public debates and excluded other issues and concerns, not least the ambivalence and complexity of prenatal testing, which this chapter aims to foreground in more detail. Importantly the pro-life lobby emerge again as a 'strange bedfellow', (chapter 2), mobilising with other groups in relation to PGD/PND. CORE, for example, has explicitly supported a number of DR campaigns and protest events on the issue of prenatal testing.

Opposition to the framing of prenatal testing as legitimate for eradicating 'serious' disease has come in particular from Disability Rights campaigners: 'The only proven cure for the vast majority of genetic conditions is ... abortion following genetic testing or embryo selection as part of IVF'(Disability Awareness in Action (DAA) 2005); 'disability rights activists ... are expressing how significant this is for them. This is ... about eradicating them' ('Mike'). They say that such tests imply *values*; who has value as a person, what traits are deemed valuable, socially acceptable or unacceptable. What traits have 'bio-value' (Waldby 2002) in our society, and which do not? DR campaigners argue that quality of life is a complex concept, challenging dominant rationales behind how it is defined, and who defines it. Trait selection or de-selection inevitably implies notions of value, and the intrinsic worth of human life: 'one of the issues that cause some disabled (and non-disabled) people particular concern: who decides what characteristics are "unwanted"?' (DAA 2005). DR campaigners have had representation on advisory bodies such as the HGC, and some have taken direct action in order to get their message heard. The DR community has a strong tradition of wishing to speak for itself; however 'organic' alliances have been made with sympathisers and supporters. HGA also addresses the emotive issues of value and worth in relation to prenatal genetic tests and screening programmes and also raises concerns about the commodification of children through PGD, framed as the 'slippery slope'.

DR accounts of human value are made clear in the following narrative of DR opposition to PND screening for Down's syndrome for women over the age of 35, which was on the point of being 'rolled out' in the UK in 2003. This text was taken from a circulated press release:

> On May 19th [2003], a group of people with Down's Syndrome and their supporters disrupted the International Down's Syndrome Screening Conference at Regents College in London. This is the first time people with Down's Syndrome have made such a protest and is a major new step in the debate about genetics, eugenics and the rights of disabled people ... Ms Souza, who is a trustee of the Down's Syndrome Association, told the doctors that she opposes Down's Syndrome screening and that people with Down's Syndrome are people not medical problems. Her speech was warmly applauded by the conference delegates.
>
> The protesters consisted of three people with Down's Syndrome, another disabled person with learning disabilities and their families and supporters. They had written to the conference organisers in advance and asked to speak, but were refused ... It is unacceptable that doctors discuss better ways of preventing people with Down's Syndrome being born, whilst excluding their voices from the debate. This runs directly counter to one of the main demands of disabled people: 'Nothing about us without us' ... This should be the start of a national debate on prenatal screening.
>
> (Souza 2003)

The protest raised important and highly emotive issues of value, worth and identity; recurring DR discourses in this domain. The lack of proper public engagement is also a key issue framed by these campaigners and by 'sustainability citizenship' groups, as well as the issue of geneticised identities in relation to genetic tests; for example how individual and group identity is shaped by genetic information provided in specific contexts, and how this shaping is being responded to – up-taken or resisted – by affected groups and individuals. This issue is discussed in more detail in chapter 6.

While it is possible to identify a 'pro and anti' clash between pro test patient groups and anti test DR groups, the more nuanced reality is an acknowledgement from all sides of complexity, ambivalence, and often intensely difficult and emotive decisions in relation to prenatal genetic testing. Thus while generally patient groups are mobilising over wanting better access to a range of genetic tests, concern is also articulated, from these same patient groups, around the implications of testing, whether adult or prenatal. Similarly, DR groups generally opposed to prenatal testing in particular on grounds of 'slippery slopes' are generally very careful not to 'point fingers' at individuals who make difficult 'choices', and may very well have or use genetic information themselves if offered it. Ambivalence and complexity are expressed by the majority of engaged individuals, around the acknowledged difficulties of 'to test or not to test'. 'Pro or anti testing' is less the 'real' debate than the framing of complexity.

you will find people within the disability community who will say, I can completely understand why a woman who has a pregnancy test and it comes up with this disease would opt for a abortion, and others who will say that's discrimination.

('Sally')

However despite the framing of complexity, DR activists in particular have framed prenatal testing in terms of eugenics.

women are saying its about having a choice ... I think that's fair enough if women really want that, but they need to understand that that is eugenics and that's what they're choosing to do; but it's not a woman's right to choose, that then becomes a women's right to take part in a genetic cull.

('Sally')

We believe that pressures to expand the use of PGD stem from existing eugenic tendencies in our society, and might potentially lead to a full-blown consumer eugenics ... we should not be complacent and expect that either the complexity of genetic determination or the invasive nature of IVF will present permanent barriers to the widespread use of PGD.

(HGA 2000)

Most disabled people do not oppose ... genetic testing – if it is part of an ameliorative therapy or the treatment of illnesses or genetic conditions. What we do oppose is eugenic cleansing carried out in the name of treatment. The price is too high for everyone.

(DAA 2005)

Genetic testing/screening, specifically at prenatal level, is thus framed by many 'prime movers' as being eugenics by the back door. Eugenics, like genocide, is an emotive word not to be bandied about. However the issue needs addressing. The cost of illness is a rationale for PND and PGD genetic testing given in a Department of Health White Paper (Dept of Health 2003). This is the classic definition of eugenics – where people's lives, and worth, are measured in economic terms, as they were in Nazi Germany: 'how much do disabled and ill people cost the State?' (Poore 2007).

The second definition of eugenics is one of de-selection on the grounds of traits seen to be of less value. On both counts, PND/PGD could thus be defined as eugenics. However Libertarian bio-ethicists (Savulescu 2001) who argue in favour of 'choice' in relation to the screening out of traits and conditions tend to also argue that eugenics is a state-enforced policy; and because trait selection is a matter of 'individual choice', then this is QED not eugenics. But others, such as HGA, argue that these tests are nonetheless developed by the state and in the case of Down's syndrome, come in the form of an opt-out screening policy. The concept of 'liberal eugenics' has been used by HGA and other campaigners to address the individualising of responsibility for prenatal tests offered by the state. Those identifying the danger of eugenics also generally say that they are not pointing fingers of blame if people (women) have prenatal tests and decide to abort foetuses, or not implant them (see chapter 7). Rather, they wish to tackle head-on the issue about where society is going.

Commercially available adult genetic testing

This second example focuses on another category of test: commercially available adult tests. The potential for commercial development of the test-as-output has been evident for some time: 'genetics is quite difficult to com-mercialise in some ways. The obvious output of genetics is the diagnostic test' ('Ian'). Chapter 4 identified how the test itself was becoming the end product; diagnostics is a highly powerful emergent industry in 'big pharma'.[9] This is resulting in an emergent, burgeoning sector selling com-mercially available 'direct to consumer' tests, triggering a significant amount of public engagement, in the UK and worldwide (GeneWatch 2009; Prainsack *et al.* 2008; *Observer* 2008). There is an identifiable public shift into 'bio-consumerism', which has been also noted by those with an interest in policy (NCoB 2003):

> we did ... a 'YouGov' survey ... done on the basis that a lot of the people who are going to potentially ... buy genetic tests will be doing so over the internet, so trying to tap into those sorts of groups.'
>
> ('Angela')

People appear to be keen to participate, constructing (or quite literally buying into the constructions of others') genetic meanings in terms of future health, security, predictability and identity. Public access to commercially available genetic test kits which claim to be able to identify an individual's predisposition to a range of adult-onset and carrier status genetic diseases, mean that the public can be seen as consumers who are targets for the test-as-product. The *availability*, especially the commercial availability, of genetic tests is a separate issue to whether these tests actually *work* or even if they do, what this means in terms of available treatment or cures, and the risks of negotiat-ing this information. Such consumer publics are potential patients; more and more 'members of the general public' could be tested for genetic conditions and co-construct themselves in terms of being part of disease communities. This may be useful information for some, especially if offered as part of services for disease communities (such as Huntington's) within the NHS. The construction of 'publics as patients' via the commercial testing sector is more contested territory, and has been the focus of much criticism from 'sustainability citizenship' prime movers such as the watchdogs GeneWatch and ETC.

A key driver for commercial companies is the potential market for such tests; it is in the financial interest of relevant companies to 'sell' them as widely as possible. For example, psychological/psychiatric conditions are the subject of commercial genetic test marketing, as this newspaper article extract highlights:

'Internet gene tests provoke alarm':

> biotechnology checks for bipolar depression and schizophrenia will soon be sold over the web, despite warnings from leading psychologists … companies including NeuroMark, Psynomics and Suregene intend to offer testing for gene variants that might increase an individual's chances of suffering bipolar depression or schizophrenia … 'These tests will only worry, confuse and mislead the public and patients', said psychiatrist Professor Nick Craddock of Cardiff University. 'There is a long way to go before we have genetic tests which may be helpful to patients. Using tests at the moment is only likely to cause harm.'
>
> (*The Observer* 2008)

The article highlights a number of key points: the rapid proliferation of commercially available tests; the increasing 'geneticisation' of complex multi-factorial diseases despite well established identified scientific complexity and uncertainty in relation to predictability (chapters 3, 6). Also key is the absence of any structured counselling; contrast this anything-goes market, with the step-by-step ethical counselling approach of familial genetic testing which is part of the UK regulatory framework (NHS 2007). This issue enrols a further issue relating to people's capacity to understand, assess, negotiate and manage risk, especially in relation to what information is provided and the way it is framed (chapters 6, 7, 8).

The extension of such 'free market' logic is seeing companies such as '23 and me' offer potential customers the opportunity to 'get the latest on your DNA with $399 and a tube of saliva'.[10] The service offers personal feedback on individual predisposition to a range of traits and conditions based on SNP analysis: 'We read more than 500,000 locations in your genome using the same analytical tools as many top research labs … '[11] Highly significantly, consumers of this product are essentially paying to hand over their bio-sample (and intellectual property of this sample) for a privately owned database, even as they are given access to the results of this sample;[12] itself a dubious benefit, as the terms and conditions point out: '23andMe Service Is For Research and Educational Use Only. We Do Not Provide Medical Advice, And The Services Cannot Be Used For Health Ascertainment or Disease Purposes'.[13] At last count, '23 and me' provided SNP test results for 112 traits and conditions with a genetic component,[14] including a list of 'usual suspects' by now familiar to the reader:

- breast cancer
- colorectal cancer
- heart attack
- multiple sclerosis
- obesity
- Parkinson's disease
- prostate cancer
- type 2 diabetes

Prime movers are voicing concerns about market-driven, consumer forms of bio-identities, an issue also raised in chapter 4 and returned to in chapter 6. Some further examples of key issue frames relating to commercially available adult testing are reliability, accuracy, stigma and discrimination. GeneWatch has focused on the question of how reliable a specific test is, especially commercially available ones, stating that the reliability of genetic information is exceptionally context-dependent, and that there is much disagreement within the scientific community about what the information at a particular locus in a gene might actually signify. Genetic information plays an important role in disease expression, in some cases more than others (such as single-gene disorders). However the genetic link is more tenuous in other cases and highly suspect in still others. Many conditions for which tests are now commercially available, such as many of the 'usual suspects' in the above list, have a very small genetic component, or the significance of the genetic component may vary in different forms of the disease, such as different types of breast cancer. There are a number of variables impacting on the reliability of genetic information in different contexts. See chapters 3, 6 and 8 for further discussion on the reliability and predictive capacity of genetic information, and the implications for the person taking the test.

Chapter 8 further develops the implications underlying the promissory discourse accruing to testing, that by understanding something about oneself, by identifying risk, these risks can be avoided. In fact, as the newspaper article on depression makes clear, the reverse is also likely – that one will feel (unnecessarily) concerned about risks one didn't know were possible, and in many cases relating to commercially available tests, which are not statistically significant. This issue led 'Peter' to state that

> I think there has to be regulation ... like a ... kitemark, British Standard. ... so that it's a standardised test that's been rigorously evaluated ... before people go off and start testing themselves. Obviously ... the hypochondriacs will do that.
>
> ('Peter')

Whether a kite-mark is enough protection for todays' potential bio-consumer is questionable.

Discrimination and stigma potentially arise in relation to testing and screening in all contexts (prenatal and adult, private and public healthcare). Specific examples are given in chapter 3 and chapter 6, in relation to potential stigma and discrimination accruing from tests offered as UK healthcare policies. For example, concerns have been raised about genetic discrimination in terms of race (Wailoo and Pemberton 2006). The potential for the misuse of genetic information accrued from commercially available tests is also an issue. Much concern is raised by 'Watchdogs' in relation to how individuals may be stigmatised if they are found to be genetically predisposed to certain conditions. The UK insurance moratorium shows how the genetics and discrimination debate is being taken seriously. This is also a concern for generally 'pro test' patient groups. Watchdogs such as CornerHouse and GeneWatch have discussed adult testing and screening in terms of potential genetic discrimination and social justice issues, such as insurance: 'With genetic screening becoming more widespread ... more people [will be] rejected by insurance companies or fail to keep up premium payments that will undoubtedly increase after 'susceptibilities' are discovered' (Sexton 2002). These issues are returned to in chapter 6, which also provides detailed discussion of the implications of testing for social justice and health policy.

Conclusion

This chapter has provided an overview of what sorts of genetic tests and screens are available, in what circumstances, and provided some snapshots of how various prime movers are framing the debates. In relation to tests and screens, specifically prenatal ones, there exists a prominent discourse of pro-life, 'versus' pro choice. However there are many other issues at stake, and polarised debates don't help publics negotiate arenas of complexity and ambivalence where many different issues, knowledge and values claims are involved and enrolled, which need to be carefully unravelled. Further, being supportive of an individual 'right' to a test does not necessarily mean that someone takes that test lightly or without awareness of the many ramifications or repercussions.

Publics who are increasingly encountering genetic tests in a variety of circumstances will need to think carefully about the differences between cases, and about how different types of test exist for different purposes. Some argue that in various ways, market-led science (the bio-economy) is driving the agenda, for example the implications of the blurring of publics, patients and bio-consumers. A further issue is how predictive/accurate 'the science' is. These uncertainties have policy implications when genetic testing is often seen as a 'good thing', generally framed through a discourse of 'choice'. This is tackled head on by 'Mike':

I just get a sense of with all of these genetic technologies which is that they will half work, they will be half right, and that in itself is almost more of a problem. If they look like they're working, they appear to be working. ... under a particular paradigm of knowledge that we have, you can put them out and you can separate the findings and you can restructure health care around them.

('Mike')

Risk, uncertainty and ambivalence in relation to testing are argued by some to be not well understood/catered for, such as the significance of interventions on people/families. For example, while there is a rapid expansion of available tests, there is evidence that counselling services are struggling to keep up with demand. Mundanely and predictably, money and resources are not sufficient for the need, even when the test is offered within an NHS framework:

> these people have a condition called Familial Hypercholesterolemia ... high cholesterol levels ... it runs in the family ... and you can be screened and offered appropriate health care ... these people were very lost and very worried because they were part of a support group but there was just no health care service in Wales for them ... what they needed [was for] the health care service to address their health care issues appropriately.

('Jane')

Critiques about the promissory discourse in the Department of Health White Paper (2003) about genetic screening and testing being offered to patients, and especially the idea of genetic screening of newborns, also arose from doctors and genetic counsellors who stated that genetic counselling services would not be able to meet the demand. Debates on the individualising of responsibility for health are also germane to the policy implications, and are discussed further in chapter 6. The complex discussions about the implications of testing taking place across the spectrum from prenatal to adult, from 'serious' to 'minor' conditions, tests predicting susceptibility rates and those identifying carrier status, issues of ownership and access, represent a time bomb of explosive future public engagement.

6 Genetic exceptionalism, health, identity and citizenship

'the genetic information is real, the meanings are constructed'

(Marks 2007)

Introduction

The final three chapters of this book address in more detail some of the issues and concepts which have been shown in the previous chapters to underpin much public discourse on human genetics. This chapter examines the concept of geneticisation, showing how people construct, and engage with, geneticised accounts of (especially) health and identity in different contexts. A key frame in much genetics discourse is the assumption, implicit or explicit, that there is something 'exceptional' or special about genetic/ genomic knowledge, and that it takes precedence over other explanations or knowledge bases. This is geneticisation, which at its most extreme can be classified as genetic hype. To understand these debates, it is important to be clear about the ways in which genetics is or is not really exceptional; this chapter aims to ensure a good definition of genetic exceptionalism and hence to disentangle some of the debates. This chapter thus first critically examines genetics' exceptional status as it is framed by specific actors in specific circumstances, and second explores how a number of these and other publics are engaging with the *construction*, and the *implications*, of 'exceptional genetics', particularly in relation to health, identity, social justice and equity, and also civil liberties and crime (chapter 3). There are important policy implications, particularly as an application of genetic exceptionalism is the formation of an ethical imperative to undertake genetic research, also framed in terms of the future (chapter 8). Section One explores the idea that there is something 'exceptional' about genetics and shows how this frequently manifests itself in three often related, and sometimes muddled ideas, which are useful to separate: genetic determinism, genetic essentialism and genetic reductionism. This is followed by an overview of genetic exceptionalism and a discussion of where it may and may not have validity as an explanation.

Section two focuses on critical public responses to geneticised accounts of health and identity. Concern about 'exceptional genetics' is a key frame in 'sustainability citizenship' prime mover discourse (chapter 1). Importantly, however, all interviewees, including those involved in the production and regulation of genetic techno-science, identified problems with genetic exceptionalism particularly in relation to health policy provision, as 'Ian' highlights:

> as you understand more and more what the genes do, you can potentially make more and more therapies. But actually ... disease prevention and healthy living is a much more cost effective way of looking after a nation's health than treating people who are ill on expensive drugs.
>
> ('Ian')

This section shows that genetic exceptionalism is often overstated and that claims of genetic exceptionalism especially in relation to health often 'frame out' other perspectives such as social justice and poverty alleviation. The assumptions of exceptional genetics can operate to exclude or mask other ways of approaching problems, such as social, cultural and economic forces, as well as issues such as inequality (Bender *et al.* 2005). Discourses of genetic exceptionalism are often linked, implicitly or explicitly, to individualist ways of explaining or looking at society. Hence exceptional genetics triggers debates about, and resistance to, notions of individualised responsibility, particularly in relation to health; this has implications for citizenship stakes-setting. Previous chapters have shown that these are issues which are consistently raised by prime movers in contexts such as drug development and genetic testing.

Section one: exceptional genetics: definitions, overviews and examples

Genetic *determinism* is a doctrine about the cause of things, in particular, human behaviour. In philosophy, the term 'determinism' generally refers to claims that human behaviour is determined by underlying physical events. This implies that, if these are understood in sufficient detail, they can be predicted, and, in the right circumstances, manipulated to desired ends. Genetic determinism is the belief that genes operate in a direct and inexorable way to produce specific outcome; this relates to Dawkins's concept of 'the selfish gene' (1976); see also Wilson's (1975)[1] definition of 'sociobiology'. This may be confined to the claim that biological systems, living things including the biology of humans, are determined by genes. It also more broadly encompasses claims that human identity, and human behaviour, is 'in the genes'. This usually focuses on individual human behaviour but may stretch to instances of group or societal behaviour. The 'exceptional' status sometimes claimed for genetics in this respect is the belief that genes have a particularly salient, or crucial, role in human biology and ultimately in human behaviour, as the ultimate basis or 'blueprint' for it. Indeed, many of the metaphors of the human genome (for example blueprint, code, book of life, or the concept of 'mapping the genome') play on genetic deterministic thinking. Such future forecasting is also discussed in chapter 8.

Developments in biology, however, especially more recent developments this century, show a far more complex picture than this, and it looks far more likely that genes play a role alongside other biological elements in a highly complex system (Rose 1997; Ho 2003). Genes clearly play a key role in biological systems, such as the creation of organs, regulating how quickly toxins are metabolised through systems, and so forth. But as previous chapters have shown, the role played by genes is variable; for example, certain 'single-gene' disorders do mean that a disease or trait will definitely be expressed. However most diseases or traits are 'common complex', 'multi-factorial' ones, where specific genes or sets of genes may play a role, or to a certain extent predispose towards disease or trait expression, but do not determine it. The idea that genes are laid down at conception, and then follow a predictable trajectory along the whole of an individual's life, has been contradicted by much research, for example showing how genes can be switched on and off[2] and affected by environmental impacts upon development (Mohrenweiser *et al.* 2003). There are various elements to these counters to genetic determinism. It may be that genes do not have such a master role in forming an individual's biology, but that other biological forces have their own crucial roles in an intricate system. Moreover, input from an organism's environment may modify the role of genes (Lichtenstein 2000). And many argue that to understand individual and social behaviour, we need to make use of psychological and social concepts; genes themselves cannot be singled out as causes of complex phenomena such as voting patterns, or the ability to play the French horn, or as the causes of many complex traits, such as intelligence (Rose 1997).

As Annette Karmiloff-Smith, Professor of Neurocognitive Development, Institute of Child Health, said at a conference in 2003:

> there's no such thing as a gene, or even a specific set of genes, for intelli-
> gence ... each gene has a number of outcomes ... paradoxically, the more
> we know about the importance of the gene, the more we realise about the
> importance of environmental influences.
> (Annette Karmiloff-Smith speaking during the Institute of Ideas Genes
> and Society conference, April 2003.)[3]

Nevertheless, deterministic elements of predictability are still rife in public commentary and speculation about genetics. This goes from the silly jokes about having the 'gene for' eating cream cakes as an excuse for being chubby, to the serious, such as speculation about finding 'genes for' criminality. Genes obviously do have a large role to play in human biology and behaviour. The challenge, in predicting, understanding and modifying, is to accurately understand that role and its place amidst other causes.

Genetic *reductionism* is the belief that complex biological phenomena can be explained completely by reference to genes. In general terms, with some important qualifiers, the identification of 'genes for' the majority of traits, conditions and diseases is a reductive means of constructing disease (Gardner 2003). Genetic reductionism is used even more ambitiously to construct accounts of human or societal behaviour. For example, some researchers have claimed that genetic differences between people incline some but not others to have so-called religious experiences (Saver and Rabin 1997). This explanation is reductionist if it claims to have understood the phenomenon entirely, without the need to introduce other concepts such as 'real' spiritual experiences, or other psychological or social phenomena that cannot be entirely explained in terms of genes.

The complexity of biological systems makes implausible a general genetic reductionism that attempts to reduce all human thought and behaviour to genetic origins. Although explaining phenomena in terms of more simple components is an extremely powerful and useful tool, there are good reasons to be wary of its overuse. Many phenomena operate as systems, where complex pathways of causation mean 'top down' approaches to explanation need to be seen alongside 'bottom up' or more systems-based and holistic approaches. According to 'Alice', this is the ' systems biology'[4] potential of genomics:

> genomics ... is dispelling that myth of a gene for this and a gene for that. It's making people look at the cell and the body as an organic whole. It's something of an ecology ... rather than ... trying to negate a disease state, actually thinking about the whole system holistically.
>
> ('Alice')

Genetic *essentialism* is the belief that genes are the essence of human or individual identity or relationships, community groupings, and of a sense of self. 'Jenny' addresses such essentialism when she says:

> your genes don't make you who you are, and there are a lot of disabled people with genetic disorders who ... articulate that extremely eloquently. But there's a big push from companies to try and convince people who aren't in that box of 'disabled person with a genetic disorder' that ... for everybody their genes make them who they are. And genes are quite a small part of biology, never mind the whole environment that you live in.
>
> ('Jenny')

Our unique DNA may be said to underlie our uniqueness as individuals (although this does not explain the example of monozygotic – identical – twins). Identity, belonging and heritability are important concepts for people as individuals and as parts of different families and communities. Genetic explanations of self and identity have a role to play in such constructions; however genetic essentialism goes beyond genetics informing a sense of identity, and underlies ideas that genetic family ties are the only, or the most, important ones between people; and/or that genetic explanations (of conditions) alone make up ones identity or self. Notions of identity are tied up in thoughts that it is vital to know who one's genetic parents are to understand one's 'true' origins and identity.

Genetic essentialism may sometimes underlie ideas that racial categories are important for notions of belonging, or notions of inferiority or superiority, or 'susceptibility' to disease (Di Chiro 2008). It may underlie general materialist views of humanity: that our essence as human beings lies in our biological being and specifically in our genomes, rather than, say, in a spiritual identity, or in more cultural or political characterisations of human achievement. Moral philosophers have long argued about what if any basis there is for treating other humans with consideration and kindness. Advocates of the notion of 'kin altruism' claim an evolutionary basis for behaviours that favour those who share our DNA (Hamilton 1964). Such genetically essentialist accounts of humanity are a standard trope of many evolutionary biologists, as this newspaper article extract highlights: 'Jean Jacques Hublin, an evolutionary biologist at the Max Planck Institute for Evolutionary Biology in Leipzig said: "Studying the Neanderthal genome will tell us what makes modern humans really human"' (*Guardian* 2009b). A more measured view might be that genetic information forms a part of who we are as individuals, as families, as communities, as humans, but that to focus too much on genetics as the essence of who we are detracts from a social locating of self and community. A very different definition of humanity was offered on BBC Radio 4's 'Thought For the Day' programme on 26 February 2009, by the Reverend Dr David Wilkinson, who said: 'the gift of relationship lies at the core of what it is to be human'.

Here is another example of genetic essentialism in operation. Because the Y chromosome is passed intact from father to son (with the exception of occasional mutations) it is possible to trace one's ancestry back through the male lineage by comparing Y chromosomes. Many have done this. Others seem to use such research to investigate notions of identity or essence. For example, many African Americans (and others) have traced ancestry back to specific areas or even tribes in Africa, and many seem to believe that this was important to their identity and gave them a sense of belonging.[5] However, this only traces one's father's father's father and beyond – only a tiny fraction of one's ancestry. One generation back, we have two ancestors. Two generations, we have four. After ten generations, or a mere two to three hundred years, we have more than one thousand. Y chromosome analysis only gives us information about one of these. In the case of the Y chromosome, this does correlate with surnames and with a major cultural way of grouping what it is to be a family. But a moment's reflection on our genetic ancestry, as opposed to our family name, should reveal this sense of belonging as a sham. Unless one has extra metaphysical beliefs about the primacy of the male line of transmission, how can this give us a sense of 'belonging'? Two immediate answers suggest themselves: one, that some people are so hungry for a sense of belonging that they will find it in whatever place they can discern meaning. Two, that we over-identify with the power of DNA to tell us about ourselves. Similarly, the Genographic Project invokes very strong frames of identity in relation to genetic heritability:

> Did you ever wonder about your most ancient ancestors?
> The Genographic Project will introduce you to them, and
> explain the genetic journeys that bond your personal
> lineage over tens of thousands of years
>
> (Genographic Project 2008)

Drawing variously on elements of genetic determinism, reductionism and essentialism, the notion of *geneticisation* thus makes claims for the exceptional nature of genetics:

> Geneticisation refers to an ongoing process by which differences between individuals are reduced to their DNA codes, with most disorders, behaviours and physiological variations defined, at least in part, as genetic in origin. It refers as well to the process by which interventions employing genetic technologies are adopted to manage problems of health. Through this process, human biology is incorrectly equated with human genetics, implying that the latter acts alone to make us each the organism she or he is.
>
> (Lippman 1991)

Geneticisation is a term first coined by Abby Lippman, a professor of epidemiology at McGill University in Canada, representing the claim that genetic aspects of a situation are highlighted to the detriment or exclusion of others. Hence, a more rounded or holistic appraisal of problems and possible solutions is bypassed. Many critics who see geneticisation as a problem consider that social and other responses to problems are in danger of being sidelined in favour of an undue emphasis on genetic causes and genetically based solutions. Further, various 'prime movers' have identified how such geneticisation can actually exacerbate health inequities (Section Two).

A kindred but older and more wide-ranging term is that of medicalisation, where social problems are subsumed into a medical model. For example, social and psychological circumstances that might give rise to a problem such as depression amongst mothers caring for young children are overlooked and the problems treated medically with drugs. Furthermore, as well as this tunnel vision, an aspect of medicalisation is that of medical 'creep': the wider the spread of medicine, the greater the power of the medical profession, and the greater the chance of medically induced (iatrogenic) problems, such as, in the above example, addiction to the drugs given to treat depression (Illich 1975). Section Two returns to the tricky landscape where identity and health collide through geneticised 'syndrome invention' and the construction of 'the patient as consumer', discussed in chapter 4 and also chapter 5.

Disability Rights (DR) activists are very alert to geneticisation as an extension of medicalisation; much DR campaign work has focused on emphasising how social attitudes to conditions need to be unpacked, rather than society seeing the conditions themselves as something 'defective'. 'Sally' outlined an important aspect of DR philosophy, which critiques this 'medical model' of disability as opposed to

> what we call a social model, a social definition of disability, which is that disability is the interaction between someone with an impairment and the rest of the world. So to us we're disabled when we meet a barrier and it's a barrier that we can't move and change that makes us disabled. The most simple manifestation of that is we'd say that somebody in a wheelchair becomes disabled when they meet a flight of stairs and can't get into a building.

While there are some detailed debates on the 'social model' within and without the DR community which warn against over-simplification of a very complex topic (Yeo 2007; Kerr and Shakespeare 2002), in general terms the DR definition of medical models versus social models of disability is very important in helping us to think in broad terms about how genetic exceptionalism potentially unfairly individualises responsibility and/or geneticises identity in ways which those with the specific genetic condition or trait themselves resist.

There are, of course, a number of important examples where 'genetic exceptionalism' can fairly said to have legitimacy in that the gene clearly has a highly important, not to say unique, function. Previous chapters have given examples such as the 'single-gene disorders', which include Cystic Fibrosis (CF), Down's syndrome, Huntington's disease, Duchenne's Muscular Dystrophy (chapter 5). There are a number of other conditions/traits where carrying the specific gene 'strongly predisposes' to expressing the condition, such as the BRCA1/2 breast cancer genes, or specific bowel cancer (BBC 2007). There are also a number of more minor genetic conditions such as cleft palate (BBC 2001) and types of deafness (*The Times* 2007) which are consistently identifiable through genetic testing (chapter 5).

Genes clearly play a role in many functions of biological systems, such as the P450 family of genes (GHR 2008) which enable the system to metabolise and detoxify chemical toxins. Many such genes are 'expressed' differently in different individuals; these individual micro-variations are known as Single Nucleotide Polymorphisms (SNPs). Chapter 4 discussed the promise of pharmacogenomics as 'personalised pharmaco' where such genomic variations or polymorphisms in typologies of traits and conditions can be identified; for example they have been identified as accounting for the fact that different individuals metabolise drugs at different rates. Such minute differences could mean the difference between life or death for individuals.

It is often argued that genetic diseases, genetic material, genetic information, or DNA itself, are exceptional in some way, and that because of this exceptional status, practice and policy needs to differ in various respects from general medical practice. A number of different arguments are advanced for genetic exceptionalism, such as that genetic diseases, and genetic information, have implications for other family members who may also have or carry the condition: hence normal notions of individual privacy and confidentiality are becoming challenged. It is argued that DNA is unique in its status in passing down biological information between generations: it relates both to individual health and identity, and to reproduction. Other claims for exceptional status are that DNA and genes play a unique role in creating and regulating biological systems; that genetic information is an especially powerful identifier of persons and hence extra caution in regard to privacy may be needed; that genetic information is unique in its role of characterising who we are as individuals and as a species, including subgroups of the population. Another claim for genetics' exceptional status is that genetic information is an especially powerful tool because of the capacity to gather it from minute samples, without the knowledge or consent of the individual.

However, it has also been argued that many features are not actually unique to DNA but shared by many other aspects of biology and of disease. For example, transmissible diseases such as syphilis and TB also have potentially weighty implications for other family members. Some of the claims are based upon biological accounts of the unique role of DNA, now known to be exaggerated or in need of modification. Martin Richards (2001) argues that the 'uniqueness' attaches more to cultural images of the special status of DNA, and that we need to distinguish 'biological' DNA from 'metaphorical' DNA.

A certain amount of genetic exceptionalism is thus scientifically/medically justifiable, but the extent to which the genetic/genomic information is exceptional is highly context-dependent. To reiterate, genes clearly play all kinds of roles in all sorts of ways; criticism of 'geneticisation' by various publics is generally not discounting this, but is rather about critically questioning discourse, policy, commercial activity and so forth which places emphasis predominantly on genetic accounts in ways which are identifiably wrong or counter-productive for a number of reasons.

Arguably, a broad consensus might be that genetic, genomic and proteomic sequencing provide genetic *information* but not necessarily *knowledge*. For example, the relationship between much gene expression and disease expression is a chicken and egg one, with huge uncertainty as to what causes gene expression. This is the case, for example, even with a 'single-gene' disorder such as BRCA1, where it is unknown why the gene 'switches on' in different people at different ages with variable prognosis, and in a significant percentage of those carrying the gene, not at all. Very importantly, just because the disease manifests at the genetic level, it doesn't mean the cause is genetic, and the issue about whether genetic damage is seen as cause or symptom of a disease or condition is key to the debates on geneticisation. The trigger for a specific gene expression could be environmental; for example, exposure to toxic waste, or smoking. A geneticised tendency to see the gene, rather than the pollution, as the problem, has significant political and policy implications for affected communities.

Even where genetic exceptionalism has scientific and medical legitimacy in terms of a diagnosis, a diagnosis is not a prognosis, for example in terms of the severity of the condition. Differential prognosis could be genetic or the result of other factors (chapter 5). Research on cures for genetic conditions focuses on looking at how the gene (or sets of genes) expresses itself. This can be really beneficial in terms of treatments, but there is not necessarily a high-tech genetic solution, or certainly not one which is easily found. For example, as regards the genetic condition Cystic Fibrosis (CF):

> there is still a lot of excitement about the gene therapy but actually what has had a staggering impact on the life expectancy of people with Cystic Fibrosis is a myriad of small increments achieved through medical research ... better antibiotics, better understanding of cross risk and better nutrition ... a thousand and one tiny improvements.
>
> ('Peter')

Genetic exceptionalism is closely linked to futures talk (chapter 8); it can distort the things we hope for and the ways we try to get them. A graphic way of illustrating the shortcomings of an over-emphasis on genetically based fixes for society's current problems is by considering a well-established genetic link with criminality: the overwhelming majority of criminals all have similarity, in that they possess a Y chromosome (they are males). Rape, burglary and other crimes, and thus the prison population, could be cut at a stroke by detecting this prenatally and offering therapeutic abortions. However, few since Valerie Solanas wrote *The Scum Manifesto* (1968) have suggested such a radical move. What this extreme example does is to show what is at stake when genetic exceptionalism is enrolled; what is needed is a proper debate about the allocation of resources and social policy provision in the 'century of the gene' (Keller 2000) or perhaps, now, the century of the genome.

Genetic exceptionalism thus has important policy implications, with regard to 'health per se' in a broad sense, and with regard to the very specific focus on a range of diseases and conditions with varying degrees of genetic causalities and how these are conceptualised; and to behaviour, identity and mental health issues. This can impact upon individuals thinking about their health and reproduction, the values of medicine, and government policy. There is also something of a tendency for discourses of genetic exceptionalism to mix up 'special cases' (see also 'saviour siblings', chapter 5) as if they had 'one size fits all' applicability, which is generally not the case. For example, whereas certain types of bipolar depression do have a significant link with specific gene expression, this example, of late championed by media personality Stephen Fry (Cardiff 2006), does not give a good account of all forms of depression, or by default imply that genetics research into depression should supersede other routes to depression prevention, treatment and cure. Cancer is often subject to such geneticisation. For example, with the discovery of the BRCA1/2 breast cancer gene, the media had a tendency to hype this as 'future promise' for all breast cancer sufferers (*Daily Mail* 2009), but the diagnosis based on the BRCA 1/2 genetic profile was only suitable for a small minority of breast cancer patients; most types of breast cancer, and cancer generally, are multi factoral.

Genetic tests for certain specific 'single-gene' disorders and chromosomal abnormalities have further consequences in terms of presenting people with choices. The fact that certain disorders are genetically linked is a 'hard' biological fact which means that it presents itself as having a certain level of legitimacy. But as discussed in chapter 5 and again in chapter 7, genetic testing and screening is a contested benefit. Debates on 'where to draw the line' are often linked to discussions of geneticisation, because potentially a large number of traits with a genetic component can be seen as a genetic disorder to be cured or screened out.

Section two: 'prime mover' responses to the implications of geneticisation

Genetic exceptionalism is thus argued to impact upon, and even to distort, policy and medical and pharmaceutical practice, as well as individual behaviour and related areas of social policy such as defining citizenship stakes (Plows and Boddington 2006). This section summarises debates which have repeatedly arisen in critical responses to frames of genetic exceptionalism. Previous chapters have shown that these counter-frames generally focus on issues of health, identity, social and environmental justice, and citizenship and public engagement. Prime movers from the 'sustainability citizenship' case study (chapter 1) in particular have been attempting to stake their knowledge claims in the context of calls for better debates and more inclusive public engagement on the policy implications of geneticisation and what is seen as being at stake:

> we definitely try to make a bigger critique ... as to why research money is going into genetics, [and not into] public health and equality and all the things which would make a much bigger difference. I think it's more difficult to make a shift in policy in that kind of area.
>
> ('Jenny')

Health: re-framing and re-locating the debates

The privileging of geneticised accounts of knowledge is of particular relevance for the issue of what constitutes health and associated strategies for health policy provision. There are also important ramifications for what diseases are looked at in policy, and how diseases are understood and tackled. Chapters 2–5 provided a number of examples of health defined in terms of promissory genetics discourses in a number of policy spaces, with important social implications such as the sorts of reproductive decisions women are now making (chapter 5). Prime movers reacting to geneticisation in a health context are trying to re-frame the debate, to re-frame the question as: 'what is health and how can we be healthy?' ('Alice'). 'Alice' makes this point clearly when she says:

> there's such a fixation these days on genomics and the gene has all the answers. Whereas really the glaringly obvious health issues, like ... malnutrition ... in mums and kids ... They are blatantly ignored. It's a hyped thing that's deflecting attention from the real health issues.
>
> ('Alice')

This re-framing of the debate enables, for example, strategies on child poverty, environmental pollution, to become as relevant as discourses on genetic exceptionalism (Wilkinson 1996; Sexton 1999). For example, life expectancy for women in Zimbabwe has dropped to an average of 35 under Mugabe's regime (BBC 2006c). There are clearly political causes for this shocking statistic, and hence political interventions can improve life expectancy (Marmot and Shipley 1996).

So what exactly is health? This is a surprisingly difficult question to answer, not to mention a complex one and this chapter does not aim to provide a definition but rather simply to highlight that many are seeking to address this broader question, particularly as a counter to geneticised accounts. Is health simply the absence of disease? There are two difficulties with this. First, it is not easy to define what a disease is. Is infertility a disease? What is a disease and what is a normal part of aging? And so on. Second, this is a very thin notion of health: surely there is more to health than simply not being ill. For instance, a carrier of a genetic condition may be healthy but worried about reproduction. Many have also worried about definitions of health that limit themselves to the physical: should health be more holistic and include psychological and social elements as well? The World Health Organisation in 1946 defined health thus:

> Health is a state of complete physical, mental and social well-being and not merely the absence of disease or infirmity.
>
> The enjoyment of the highest attainable standard of health is one of the fundamental rights of every human being without distinction of race, religion, political belief, economic or social condition.
>
> (WHO 1946)

'Sustainability citizenship' prime movers directly address the issue of what constitutes health, and QED what types of interventions will bring it about.

> the organic movement ... has a very strong concept of health, that health is something that exists in the whole system ... whereas when you look at the pharmaceutical industry, ... you don't have health as a concept you have disease ... and you're constantly battling that disease rather than starting from and building up health. And ... the geneticisation of medicines just goes further ... we're not concentrating on how do we build good health, what is a healthy person? ... We're asking what is an unhealthy person and ... how do we handle all of the defects.
>
> ('Mike')

To articulate such concerns about geneticised health strategies is *not* to be oppositional, to the point of dismissing out of hand, scientific claims about potential cures and treatments for (serious) disease accruing to the applied use of human genetics information and associated knowledge claims in specific contexts. People who are critical about the geneticisation of health are generally not oppositional to the basic idea, that genetic information, and applications derived from that genetic information (e.g. drugs) could have a positive impact on the health of global populations generally and specific 'disease communities' in particular. What is being critiqued is the predominant emphasis on geneticised accounts of health, perhaps especially the mixing up of damage to genes seen as being a cause, or a symptom of, disease/condition expression, and the implications this has for health and social policy. As the feminist academic Di Chiro points out, 'Genetic reductionism oversimplifies ... the real causes of disease' (2008: 228). It also impacts on what policy interventions are decided upon. Similarly, Blaxter (2004) has suggested that a dominant individualised discourse leads to individualised accounts of health and illness causation.

Re-framing the debates on health away from geneticised accounts enables health to be situated within many of the 'bigger picture' issues which communities, social movements, and also national and global governance are concerned about. These issues, central to the environmental justice movement (Di Chiro 2008) and following Barry (2005); referred to throughout the book in terms of 'sustainability citizenship', can be seen as forms of 'preventative health provision'; although importantly, this is *not* to reduce all issues raised by 'sustainability citizenship' actors to debates about health. These issues flow from the micro level of pollution impacts on a specific community, through to global concerns – for example war, climate change, and the effects on populations. 'Global civil society' (Eschle and Stammers 2005; Ford 2003) approaches to 'sustainability citizenship' goals range from the political/policy-orientated Sustainable Development summits of 1992 and 2002, which involved many NGOs as stakeholders (UN Wire 2002), to the much more grassroots-orientated, self-initiated convergences of campaign groups through events like the World Social Forum and grassroots networks such as the international campaign network the People's Health Movement. Broadly, peace, anti nuclear, environmental, and 'anti globalisation' social movements across several decades have all had much to say about health; for example making explicit links between capitalism, environmental degradation and pollution, and health (McMurtry 1999). For some overviews and introductions of relevant social movements and protest activity, see Mies and Shiva (1993), Shiva (1989), Barry (2005), Plows and Boddington (2006); Plows (2008c); Ainger *et al.* (2003); Routledge (2003); Welsh (2000); Chesters and Welsh (2006), Sen *et al.* (2004).

Such campaigners argue that in relation to health, geneticised accounts can hide social causes and social solutions, relegating the influence of social justice, equity and environment to barely heard background noise. An example of recent discussion on genetic causes for health problems is obesity. Many studies have discussed obesity as a socially produced phenomenon with social justice implications (Goodman and Adler 2007). However, media stories on research which identifies a 'gene for' obesity (BBC 2008b, 2008d) do not tend to locate such genetic accounts in a social context. It is likely that such a 'gene for', even if this genetic link is shown to be replicable in later studies, will be like the examples of BRCA 1/2 breast cancer or a specific form of bipolar depression given earlier; that is, only true in certain cases of obesity. Such a focus on the gene overall threatens to take our eye off the ball. Parents walking their children to school and getting them to eat more vegetables are helping their kids be healthy, and not to be obese. Of course such discourses and the actors who frame them are not incompatible with those looking at the genetic basis of diseases, but there is a tendency to privilege the geneticised accounts on the basis of its 'future promise' (chapter 8).

It is far from just 'sustainability citizenship' prime movers who identify such concerns. Those involved with the science as producers and regulators of it also express caution regarding geneticised accounts of disease and potential interventions:

> However once you then start talking about therapies you shouldn't be blinded by the genetics. So for example a lot of investment now is going into ... smoker's cough, bronchitis ... [but] instead of investing huge amounts of money to find a genetic predisposition or find drugs to treat it, the basic treatment is don't smoke.
>
> ('Ian')

> [we are] very aware of the socioeconomic factors involved in health ... you are more likely to die younger if you earn under a certain amount of money ... those facts are actually pretty well established, and what a number of the members [of the HGC] have raised is, ok we've got this focus on genetics, but what about ... decent diet ... decent maternal health will quite often potentially have much better health outcomes to

the child than looking at genetic predispositions, which we don't currently have much information on.

('Angela')

Epidemiology (Davey-Smith and Ebrahim 2005; Davey-Smith *et al.* 2005) provides a potential space where balanced genetic discourse and social justice-orientated health policy can 'crosstalk' (Bucchi 2004), for example through a social policy application of toxicogenomics (Christiani *et al.* 2007) – the study of how toxins impact on the genome – or, as discussed in chapter 3, via studies developed through the UK Biobank data. An important socially and politically focused epidemiological account of the impacts of asbestos on Indian women workers has been undertaken by the Indian physicist Qamar Rahman. More recently, she has undertaken research on the potential impacts of nanoparticles, making important comparisons politically, environmentally and at the level of individual (genetic/genomic) health damage, between asbestos and nanoparticles, providing important pointers for how to conduct politically and socially located epidemiological research which incorporates genetic/genomic information (Rahman 2008).

Where people live has a huge influence on health (cures, treatment, prevention, predictability). For example, postcodes can tell us a lot about people's life expectancy; people living in postcodes in areas of Scotland, and parts of East London, have significantly lower life expectancies than the average for the UK (*The Times* 2008c). Such a 'human geography' locates people in their environments in relation to concepts of health, and also community and identity (Savage and Burrows 2007). This raises some clear inferences; that in terms of social policies for health, postcodes are probably a more reliable predictor of health and life expectancy than gene codes. This message is being transmitted loudly, not just by genetic 'watchdogs' and social justice campaigners, but also, for example, by grassroots UK GPs. As a GP writing in the *Financial Times* about the UK Biobank said:

> The question, from my position as a GP, is what we will do with all this new [genetic] information once we have it. ... From my side of the desk, poverty, loneliness and social exclusion seem to be the biggest determinants of ill health.
>
> (*Financial Times* 2009)

Geneticisation thus often has the effect of *dislocating* the social and political landscapes of the poor, whose environments tend to be more unhealthy and who have fewer social opportunities and correspondingly more unhealthy lifestyles. Given a background of deprivation, stress and lack of opportunity, people are 'predisposed' to be more unwell, more prone to obesity, to smoke, to drink (Stafford and Marmot 2003). Focusing on susceptibility and predisposition to illness in terms of genetics, can be a means of blaming the victim. The health framing of human genetics in terms of 'choice' (chapter 7) and individualised responsibility and also 'duty' – what 'good citizens' ought to do, how they ought to live – can be seen as particularly unfair when health is located, as it ought to be, in a socio-economic, political landscape which takes account of people's environments and social circumstances.

Geneticisation, individualised responsibility and citizenship

This section develops prime mover concerns about the impacts which geneticisation has or could have on citizenship stakes. Debates about the nature and constituency of citizenship within Science and Technology Studies (STS) are linked to debates on public engagement, expertise and knowledge production; see Irwin (1995), Irwin and Michael (2003), in particular their discussions of 'scientific citizens' who are mobilising over bio-technology. Political theorists and other academics with an interest in 'green' politics have developed a conceptualisation of citizenship which focuses on issues of social justice in an age of globalisation, where environmental risks, social inequities and attendant health risks, are generally borne by the global poor (Fischer 2000; Dobson 2003, 2006; Hayward 2005, 2006; Beck 1995; Di Chiro 2008; Rahman 2008). Barry (2005) has defined this as 'sustainability citizenship'.

'Bio-citizenship,' as explicated by Rose and Novas (2004), represents an important example of the many versions of citizenship currently under discussion. The notion of bio-citizenship arises from long established debates around bio-politics (Rabinow 1996), as well as the historical development of various conceptions of citizenship. Rose and Novas (2004: 440) make a general claim that 'specific biological presuppositions, explicitly or implicitly, have underlain many citizenship projects, shaped conceptions of what it means to be a citizen, and underpinned distinctions between actual, potential, troublesome and impossible citizens'. Citizens, they argue, may be 'made up' from above by governments' particular practices that relate to corporeality or biology in some way. And biological notions have in the past, and increasingly so, shaped citizens' self-understanding (Rose and Novas 2004: 441). Rose and Novas draw on certain key examples of the empowered, informed patient-as-consumer; an engaged, mobilising actor in the bio-economy and engaging with health issues and bioscience. There is no doubt that this is an important emergent social reality. However arguably, a framing of 'bio-citizenship' reifies the stakes; locking into place the notion that the biology, the genetics, is the core issue 'in the frame' when citizens engage.

Rose and Novas have discussed bio-citizenship in terms of an individualised, 'genetic' responsibility to 'know and manage the implications of one's own genome' (2004: 141). Such a 'responsibility' could relate not only to one's own health, but also reproductive 'choices' one might make (chapters 5, 7). This is not simply related to prenatal screening and testing. Will women in the future be blamed for not eating correctly for their baby's genotype, never mind whether or not they can afford it? In Plows and Boddington (2006), this vaunted genetic 'responsibility' in Rose and Novas's (2004) account of bio-citizenship was critiqued as a dis-located account of citizenship, which frames out clearly relevant social and environmental justice variables. The reductionist focus on the biological may act to obscure the economic and other forces at play; and in turn may then act to obscure the power flows that help to make up categories as biological or otherwise, and hence help to influence strategies for action. With regard to citizenship, there is a world of difference between citizens freely mobilising in relation to bio-technology, and 'citizens' actually being manipulated – 'bio-labelled' – by the giants of bio-technology to their own ends of increasing their economic and commercial power.

Key to citizenship debates are notions of rights, duties and responsibilities; what these might consist of, and who has the power to define them. These issues have been consistently raised by 'prime movers', concerned about the power relations and values which are shaping potential citizenship roles in the arena of human genetics. Concerns have been raised about the individualising of responsibility; the issue of 'blaming and framing', especially in relation to health. Questions about citizenship entitlements and duties bring to the fore issues of equality and fairness; how can those in deprived circumstances be seen as responsible for their health when they are denied social opportunities? Accounts of sustainability citizenship consistently draw attention to issues of poverty and inequity in the context of health policy and potential duties of citizens. A key concern is who has the power to advance specific notions of duty in relation to human genetics and bioscience. It has been argued explicitly by some that we may even have a 'moral duty' to genetically enhance our children (Savulescu 2004). How far is this a step towards saying that some people should not reproduce at all? There are important debates to be had here about what it is to contribute to society, what it is to be a citizen; if your life is a financial cost, does this imply that your life has no value? The bio-ethicist John Harris (2005) has also recently invoked the notion of 'moral duty', arguing that

> Biomedical research is so important that there is a positive moral obligation to pursue it and to participate in it.
>
> (Harris 2005)

There are a number of concerns relating to Harris's claim. For instance, there are medical risks attached to some of these potential duties. Further, the (unequally distributed) risks and burdens on individuals should be taken into account in assigning such duties. Also needed is a clear and accurate analysis of how and why a particular alleged duty is needed to accomplish specific benefits; themselves unevenly distributed, and often contested.

Altruism and claims invoking 'the public good'[6] are inherent in regulatory and other discourses which advocate citizen participation in biomedical research (chapters 2, 3). Such discourses – 'giving something back' – appeal to publics, and work well in relation to blood and organ donation. These ideas, ideals, meld synergistically with desires for disease treatment and cure; concerns about health and altruistic notions of participating in society combine to produce strong accounts that citizen participation in such research is a 'public good' which can be achieved through responsible evaluation of risks and benefits. This appears unproblematic until one starts to unpack the values, and risks, inherent in specific contexts where these citizenship 'duties' or altruistic 'choices' are manifesting, such as genetic screening (chapter 5) or egg 'donation' (chapter 2). It is also important to consider how exactly citizens are exhorted to various responsibilities and acts of altruism. Notions of altruism, duties and responsibility are linked to an underlying framework of values and goals. An action can only be a duty, a responsibility, or altruistic if it is a benefit; but benefits are disputed, and benefits in relation to medicine and bio-technology are no exception. Who is benefiting, and upon which citizens do any associated burdens fall?

Chapters 4 and 5 discussed how the 'bio-economy' as a promissory discourse was pushing a certain construction of health and an accompanying type of healthcare (Birch 2006). Watchdog prime movers such as 'Mike' talked about how the drive for profit was fuelling market-led constructions of health and identity, for example bio-consumers participating in the co-construction of syndrome creation with 'big pharma'. Campaigners and academics are arguing that the bio-economy interacts with geneticisation, acting to produce and promote a product-based account of health, achievable via consumption. Health can be marketed as an outcome of a specific product or service; we could be advised on how to 'eat right for our genotype'. This has strong links to individualised responsibility for health and citizenship accounts; while some are 'blamed and framed', others may be seen as 'good citizens' because they are bio-consumers, taking 'genetic responsibility'.

Individualised responsibility for health is a social and political position, and such individualising of health is inherent in much UK government discourse[7] (for example in relation to obesity (*The Times* 2008b; BBC 2008c)). To reiterate, concerns about genetic exceptionalism primarily relate to the reframing of social problems as individual genetic ones. In an important US example, Di Chiro (2008) describes how the remit of the Environmental Genome Project (EGP 1997) is undertaking research on the identification of single nucleotide polymorphisms (SNPs) – micro-genetic variations – which may render certain populations more 'susceptible' to toxins. The specific research focus is to identify whether low-income ethnic groups living near highly polluting facilities are 'genetically susceptible' to having adverse reactions to the pollution they are living in. While the EGP states that this study will be important in identifying environmental factors which are triggering this disease, Di Chiro's analysis is that in practice 'the EGP ... represents the emergence of the geneticization or molecularization of the environmental health sciences and of public health policy' (2008: 221). In highlighting how in practice the EGP's emphasis is on identifying individual genetic variances, rather than focusing attention on the environmental causes of this ill health – the pollutants and toxins which these communities are affected by – Di Chiro identifies a double-whammy of unfairness. Those suffering the effects of the polluting environments they live in are being blamed and framed as 'genetically responsible' for their own ill health. This has major environmental and social justice implications in terms of policy:

> The idea of inherent genetic susceptibility to environmental illness and the identification of the genetically at-risk individual or sub-population makes sense only if it is accepted that environmental pollution is a given ... and inevitable component of modern society. Ultimately, this approach to environmental health policy is about placing the responsibility for ameliorating risk squarely on the shoulders of the *individual* and shifts the focus away from government responsibility and corporate accountability.
>
> (Ibid: 227)

With rather telling implications for the remit of the UK Biobank discussed in chapter 3, even a project such as the EGP, which purportedly aims to understand gene–environment interactions, is so focused on the genetics that it frames out the environmental catalyst, and pays no attention to the political issues surrounding why ethnic minority communities are living in such circumstances in the first place. There are disproportionately high rates of low income communities of colour living next to a polluting facility such as a waste incinerator or an oil refinery, and disproportionately higher incidence and mortality rates of environmental illnesses amongst these groups. There are also clear concerns about how such genetic exceptionalism could be a form of reinforced discrimination against certain (ethnic and other) groups; identifying ethnicity in terms of 'the susceptibility gene for' is beside the point; it is identifiably people of colour who are living on the margins of society, and this is a political issue, not a genetic one. Similarly, research has shown that aboriginal Australians often resist genetic explanations for their health problems on the grounds that this hides the historical and cultural causes (Anderson *et al.* 2007).

It is not simply marginalised ethnic and low income communities which are suffering the 'blaming and framing' effects of geneticisation; the issue has the potential to impact in the workplace, where genetic screening could identify people 'susceptible' to pollution which might impact on any health claims they might make or even whether they get the job in the first place.[8]

> A lot of the research is ... on the idea of being able to identify the minority of people who are susceptible to cancer, say, when exposed to certain chemicals. And it sounds great in theory ... but in practice it's totally over estimating the predictive value of the test, and targeting individuals rather than making the workplace safe for everyone.
>
> ('Jenny')

'Jenny' identifies two important components of such geneticisation; first, how viable the test is in any case; and second, the social justice/social policy implications of targeting the individual; geneticisation dis-locating the individual from the social, political and environmental context.

Genetic exceptionalism and identity

In Section one some accounts of genetic essentialism and their impacts on identity were given, such as genetic heritability and belonging, for example. Identity is heavily contested territory, and the construction of genetic identities has been shown to be problematic (chapters 4 and 5). Genetic information is impacting on constructions of identity as individuals, groups and communities respond in various ways to the genetic meanings they construct themselves or uptake from others' constructions. Publics are embracing or rejecting these genetic accounts of identity, sometimes both at once. The emergence of social groups engaging with genetics genomics has led to an important definition of 'biosocialities' (Rabinow 1996). Many people, in many ways, are mobilising over issues relating to biology in one form or another and constructing and defining their identity through it, at least in part. But geneticised accounts of identity are problematic because they can obscure other accounts of self and identity. The construction, maintenance and defence of identity is complex. Disability Rights provides a clear example of identity fragmentation in this context. Someone diagnosed with a specific syndrome could identify as a member of a patient group wanting cures; or as a member of a disability rights group mobilising over access to treatments and a range of social provision. Such an individual could see their syndrome as core to their identity, or reject the centrality of a biologically informed construction of their own identity. They may hold, or feel strongly antagonistic to some of these positions, and/or ambivalent about some or all of them. The core issue here is to recognise the complexity and ambivalence surrounding any construction of identity and of related citizenships; identities are multiple and also fluid.

Further, such geneticised accounts of self and identity are constructed in specific circumstances, which can be highly political; it is important to understand the economic, political and social context which shapes the conditions under which an online browser can order a test which (spuriously) identifies her as 'genetically predisposed' to depression. 'Watchdog' campaigners such as 'Mike' have identified the bio-economic and political forces behind such 'syndrome invention', or 'bio-consumption' patterns (chapter 4). 'Bio-consumers' buying 'bio-products' online and constructing themselves in terms of genetic predispositions is a social phenomenon triggered by market forces and developments in globalised communication strategies, and has as much to do with these sorts of social forces as with any account of innate biological identity.

A related criticism of geneticisation and medicalisation of identity is that these definitions of identity and self (shyness, for example, or tendencies towards depression) are generally social constructs and social issues, and that genetic explanations are reductionist and essentialist explanations of self which leave out other important accounts. Much prime movers' 'bio-subjectivities' critical discourse of geneticisation and medicalisation relates to the rejection of the bio-label in terms of their own identity. This is combined with a critique of the ways in which geneticised identity construction is being formed in specific social, political and economic spaces.

Bio-discrimination and stigma are also important consequences of geneticised identities. Chapter 3 discussed how three out of four black men aged 15–34 are now on the UK police DNA database (NDNAD). As, until the December 2008 EU Human Rights ruling (ECHR 2008), an individual only had to be arrested, not charged, to be on NDNAD, it is thus likely that 'institutional racism' within the police force has led to a skewed sample collection, which could, in a worst case scenario, suggest that black men are more 'genetically predisposed' to commit crime.

The question of geneticised identity construction is interrelated with accounts of health and social justice, evidenced through the 'susceptibility genes' example given above. This is a clear example of how geneticised accounts are affecting social realities and accounts of identity. Specific groups of people – ethnic groups defined as 'genetically susceptible' – have little choice but to react defensively in the terms set out by more powerful others, namely the EGP, who are framing the debate in terms of genetics. The affected groups are practically forced to react in ways which may further co-construct and reify their identity in ways in which they would prefer not to have it framed. People may not want to have their identity framed through a genetic lens, i.e. whether they are 'susceptible' to adverse reactions to specific types of pollution, or are 'genetically predisposed' to have a certain reaction. They may not wish their identity to be constructed genetically and they may even refute the viability of the science base on its own terms. But powerful actors, exercising certain knowledge claims, have made the science matter in terms of how people's identities are constructed and how they have to respond to these identity constructions. Concepts like bio-sociality and bio-citizenship need to pay more attention to the political stakes involved with geneticised identity construction (such as being 'genetically susceptible' to pollution) by powerful elites.

Conclusion

This chapter has shown that while genetics and genomics clearly play important roles in the creation and maintenance of our biological systems, and can inform our sense of self, geneticisation over-privileges this role and reifies accounts of health and identity. For example, damaged or 'mutated' genes or DNA may be the symptom, not the cause, of disease. We have seen how in certain political and policy contexts issues of environmental justice and equity, far from being framed into sharper focus through the science of genetics, are often put further outside of the frame of reference by discourses of geneticisation. This needn't be the case, and this is essentially at the heart of 'sustainability citizenship' concerns about geneticised discourses on health and the implications for publics (citizens). Many are calling for a re-framing of debates away from geneticisation, and for better participatory democracy to enable this to occur. As Di Chiro points out, '[E]nvironmental justice activists ... contest the flawed logic of genetic reductionism [which] forecloses on and erodes commitment to solving environmental problems that are the result of social and economic injustices, *not* faulty genes' (2008: 234). These are the types of debates about human genetics which need to be developed; they are central to the discourses of many prime movers whose narratives are given in this book, but in many current human genetics debates they are only faintly heard above the noise of geneticisation. Better debates can be had, which enable better 'crosstalk' between perspectives. Picking up the baton on this theme of how to best conduct debates, the next chapter looks at how many human genetics debates have been framed in terms of choice and consent and in what contexts, and how different publics have engaged with these concepts. The chapter argues that, like geneticised accounts of health and identity, frames of choice and consent have a tendency to reify debates and exclude or marginalise other perspectives.

7 Informed consent, individual choice

Introduction

Chapters 2–5 provided contextualised examples which showed how the concepts of choice and consent are central to how human genetics debates are framed. Choice and consent are key frames in the donation, selling or trade in bio-material such as DNA and human eggs (chapters 2, 3). They are key frames in debates on genetic testing and screening, for example the use of PGD and PND (chapter 5), and are also central to debates on participation in drugs and biomedical procedures trials and also access to a range of bio-products (chapters 4, 5). We have seen that these are terms which are constructed, used and also contested by different publics, both in terms of what these 'choices' and 'consents' signify, and in terms of how the concepts themselves measure up as ways of framing the debate. For example here is 'Angela' talking about prenatal screening: 'some people think screening is all about eugenics, so you have to … address those sorts of concerns, and balance it out with other issues like informed choice'. This represents a self-identified 'balanced' view from a civil servant. But how balanced is this 'for or against' framing? Arguably, it frames those voicing concerns about eugenics as being 'anti choice'.

There are other social contexts where concepts of choice and consent are found and these inform, and in turn are informed by, the development of discourses in the sphere of genetics and related bioscience. This again highlights how 'debates on human genetics' are debates about social life more generally. Informed consent, for example, is a complex and contentious subject in relation to other bio-ethical issues of bodily autonomy such as end of life. The concept of 'presumed consent' recently discussed in the UK as a feature of an 'opt-out' approach to organ donation (Dept of Health 2008b), is a discourse which could be utilised in other bio-ethics contexts such as human genetics ones.

Defining and unpacking these words is important, especially as they can mean different things to different people in different circumstances; they are not value neutral and hence the use of, and challenges to, these terms and what they signify, is a very significant aspect of human genetics debates.

Further, especially as the two terms are often used together when people are talking about a specific thing – for example, the use of PGD – it is important to identify the difference between the idea of choice as a preference, and informed consent as a bio-ethical principle with legal implications. There is a tendency for discourses on 'choice' and 'informed consent' to blur together in public discourse, including in governance settings. UK policy makers and regulators in particular are using (and defining) informed consent and also individual choice in specific arenas. They have a key role in terms of setting the framework for public consultation and debate. The HFEA uses informed consent as a key term in relation to egg 'donation' (chapter 2). The National Screening Committee (NSC) has multiple documents relating to screening procedures, and interestingly the term informed choice appeared in a web-mounted document summarising its criteria whereas the term informed consent was absent.[1] As discussed in chapter 2 and chapter 3, those involved in the collation of bio-samples, such as the UK stem cell bank, are themselves involved in defining informed consent criteria. The Human Genetics Commission (HGC) discusses informed consent and also makes significant use of the term 'choice'; an important 2004 HGC public consultation document on PGD and PND was entitled 'Choosing the future' (HGC 2004). Bio-ethics stakeholders and related ethical advisory bodies such as Nuffield also refer to choice, as well as consent, as a key term.

Section one examines the use of informed consent in specific circumstances, and using examples from chapters 2–5, shows ways in which it is defined, used, and also challenged, by different prime movers. For example, feminists have queried whether the definition and use of informed consent in relation to egg donation in the UK is too narrow a concept fully to do justice to the range of issues at stake when such procedures are being considered. Informed consent in a medical context is a specific bio-ethical principle, developed in relation to patients (Herring 2006). It is an established aspect of procedures in human genetics which involve people, for example, as donors of bio-material, or as potentially undertaking a genetic test. Informed consent protocols are being developed in highly context-specific ways concurrent with developments in the biomedical field; for example, informed consent criteria in relation to DNA donation to the UK Biobank have been co-constructed as the Biobank developed through its pilot stages (chapter 3).

Section two provides situated examples of how, when, why, where and by whom 'choice' is used, responded to and challenged. 'Choice' is a term frequently used in tandem with, or as a substitute for, informed consent, in similar contexts relating to people's interactions with human genetics and bioscience. 'Choice' is consciously used as a key means of framing debates for specific prime movers, notably 'pro research' patient groups and 'pro science' lobby groups. People talk about informed, and individual choice; they also talk about a 'right to choose' and about 'freedom of choice'. It is also very important to analyse the words 'informed', 'individual', 'right' and 'freedom' which often accompany the terms consent and choice. All these words have significant implications and inherent values attached. They can have political resonances; for example, the term 'freedom of choice' was very much a tenet of the Blairite era (Blair 2007). There are important parallels between the discussion about individualised responsibility for one's own health (chapter 6) and the idea of an 'individual right to choose'. There is an implication of citizenship as an individualised condition in many of these terms. The idea of people as citizens having a 'right' to make highly individualistic 'choices' enrols a specific model of society.

Section one: informed consent

Contemporary bio-ethics has engaged with notions of informed consent in a great deal of detail and in many settings, such as 'end of life' (Dept of Health 2008a). Informed consent in medicine is well established as a bio-ethical, regulatory and legal principle, related to the rise of patient autonomy and protection as the prominent value in bio-ethics, and also related to legal cover for the medical practitioner. The terms of informed consent are actually very broad, despite the legal requirement; all that is required is that the patient 'must understand in broad terms the nature of the procedure which is intended' (Herring 2006: 83).

Informed consent forms are now a routine part of patient care, for example when a patient undergoes an operation. Informed consent thus provides a particular benchmark for research ethics, and is being rolled out as an ethical cornerstone of a rising number of genetics and biomedical procedures. Some of these are relatively well established, such as with regard to familial screening for heritable genetic conditions and associated genetics counselling (Featherstone *et al.* 2006; Clarke 1998) while others are works in progress, such as the development of protocols for the procurement, storage and use of bio-samples.

Despite the laudable aim of wishing to provide patient-centred models of medical practice, which, informed consent at its most aspirational arguably is, there are several significant concerns about the actual practice of informed consent, such as that it is not necessarily desirable; that it is unrealisable in practice, and thus that there is a 'myth' of informed consent – is it there merely as a tick in the box? There is often an assumption that the assurance of individual consent is sufficient to address any ethical or policy concerns; informed consent as a signed piece of paper is often viewed as 'enough' for ethics (Corrigan 2003) and certainly in terms of legal cover for the medical practitioner; if someone consents to something, it must be okay for a doctor or someone to do it to them. A question increasingly being asked as informed consent is used in settings such as the sourcing of bio-material and genetic testing, is whether the concept and its remit is fit for purpose. Does it function well enough to cover the range of issues at stake; what is it that people are being informed about, by whom, and in what circumstances?

Some argue that by focusing on autonomy and individual risk, informed consent often leaves out the social and political context and also what is tacitly recommended; the clinic setting, the availability of specific applications such as PGD and how these have been made available (chapter 5). This was addressed specifically in relation to the 2006 HFEA 'donating eggs' consultation (HFEA 2006) in an academic feminist workshop (chapter 2). The HFEA's framing of the 'donating eggs' issue in terms of informed consent came in for major criticism on several counts. The workshop discussed the politics of this 'informed-ness'; what is it deemed necessary to inform women about?

> The consultation should have clarified precisely when, how and in what circumstances women would be asked to donate their eggs for research to ascertain whether 'informed consent' is at all feasible. Women are most likely to be approached to provide some of their ova for research when they are seeking or undergoing IVF treatment ... asking women to donate their eggs whilst they are concentrating on managing the IVF process is problematic. We question, therefore, what 'informed consent' would mean in this context.
>
> (Plows *et al.* 2006: 4)[2]

There are also concerns about the viability of the globalised spread of Western models of informed consent as a legal framework, for example in India in relation to IVF. In this context, informed consent has been criticised as being a concept 'exported' (Riessman 2005) from an alien culture which doesn't address the specific cultural needs of the women in particular circumstances. It may provide legal cover for the medical practitioners involved, but is it fit for purpose?

Further, it is questionable what informed consent means to individuals when their incentive for participation is financial and hence risks are more likely to be discounted. In drugs trials where healthy volunteers are paid to test new drugs, the procedures which have arisen in order for the trial to get to this stage have undergone highly rigorous vetting, where the protocols for each trial are assessed by an independent ethics committee, operating in the UK under the terms of the Medicines for Human Use (Clinical Trials) Regulations (Dept of Health 2004a). The trial is the end point of years of work and rigorous stages of testing, and few drugs actually get to the clinical trial stages. Volunteers must give informed consent to the trial and these criteria are vetted. All these safeguards were in place in March 2006 when the TGN1412 trial went wrong, causing six healthy male volunteers to become critically ill. The £1,100 fee for taking part in the trial was one of a number of standard inducements offered to enlist volunteers, whose sole reason for participation was financial. All signed informed consent forms, but as *The Daily Telegraph* put it, *'Volunteers never think it will happen to them'* (*Daily Telegraph* 2006).

An individual's 'informed consent' can affect others whether they wish it or not, for example in a situation of genetics testing for familial inheritance, where the disclosed results of person A being tested can have implications by default for other family members. Conversely, an individual testing positive for a genetic test which has implications for other family members, may not wish other family members to know that they have had this test themselves and tested positive for whatever condition or trait the test was for. If a patient who has tested positive for a serious heritable genetic condition, with implications for other family members, does not give consent for other family members to be told, this produces a quandary for medical practitioners. The perceived need to pass on information to other family members conflicts with an individual's right to privacy, and at some point this issue may have to be dealt with through the establishing of a legal precedent (Hope 2004).

There also gaps in informed consent as practice, where policy or law has not yet been established in terms of standardised protocols. Chapter 3 discussed how developments in some areas such as DNA databases make broad assumptions about the acceptability of certain practices, such as patenting, which are not specifically mentioned and thus bypass consent. Chapter 2 and chapter 3 both discussed how research uses of donated bio-material (DNA, tissue, eggs) change over time in ways it is difficult or even impossible to predict, meaning that informed consent given for the use of donated material in specific circumstances can become obsolete. The implications of this have been to make informed consent criteria so broad – for example the UK Biobank ask for DNA samples 'for research purposes' – as to beg the question, why bother asking for it in the first place? In relation to DNA sample donation, 'Jenny' noted that

> it depends on the terms and the consent that [biobanks] sought in the first place. But there definitely can be things going on that people don't know about. Certainly patenting without people's knowledge ... And most of the researchers say well if its anonymised, you can do what you like, really. Well with ethical 'creep'.
>
> ('Jenny')

Of course, issues such as patenting of bio-samples will matter to some people more than others, and to others not at all; but such 'ethical creep' is an important issue and is demonstrably having a negative impact on the trust relationship between publics as potential donors, and those who own the donated bio-material such as the Wellcome Biobank. Clearly, informed consent does not cover all the bases, and there is patchy, or even non-existent, addressing of informed consent governance gaps in a variety of different circumstances. For example, GeneWatch note that the NHS's proposals in its 2004 white paper to (as GeneWatch put it) 'barcode babies' soon after birth, may breach the child's individual right to give or withhold informed consent (GeneWatch 2004: 5). Importantly, consent – informed or otherwise – is completely bypassed when a DNA sample is taken from someone who is arrested and charged (chapter 3).

Finally, in practice it is hard to cater for the individual in context, e.g. adjusting to what each individual person wants or needs to know. There are problems with the sheer amount of information around, which can confuse people at point of contact. Risk information and risk calculations may not be well communicated or understood, or even ignored, for example risk calculations of healthy people undertaking drugs trials for financial reward are likely to be skewed. In relation to IVF, Parry (2006) notes confusion about what consent was given, in clinic settings, when women are in situations of high stress. This was also an issue in relation to the conditions under which women might donate eggs for cloning research (chapter 2), and in relation to whether women clearly understood what their eggs would be used for:

> There is a lack of clarity regarding the type of research for which the eggs would be used. The main anticipated use would be for research directed at understanding, treating or curing conditions and diseases and not at treating infertility. But this distinction is not sufficiently clear in the consultation document. Making this point clear is important if women are to be fully informed in making their decisions about the donation process.
>
> (Plows *et al.* 2006: 6)

There are problems also with uncertainty, meaning that informing people about uncertain outcomes and how to navigate, how to calculate, the risks and benefits of whether or not to take a test, is not easy. Issues here include the limits of predictability, even for 'single-gene' disorders; a genetic diagnosis is not a prognosis (chapter 5). Further, genetic information can be simply misleading, such as the 'at risk' status of individuals who buy commercially available genetic tests of dubious utility (GeneWatch 2007; Wallace 2008b).

Of course it is important to emphasise individual capacity to navigate through complex information, which people do on a daily basis in many situations and are increasingly encountering in relation to human genetics. Certain individuals, such as patients, will acquire expertise through living with their conditions, for example, and thus are very able to give 'informed consent' in terms of understanding their condition and issues of risk accruing to different possible interventions – as Kerr *et al.*'s (1998a, b) examples of patients with 'embodied expertise' demonstrate. This is also important for children:

> When is a child old enough to understand and give consent to complex medical treatment? ... Priscilla Alderson, Professor of Childhood Studies at the Institute of Education, says ... that even very young children could give or withhold informed consent to medical treatment.
>
> (*The Guardian* 2008b)

However, this does not mean by default that *all* patient groups, individuals and so on develop such capacity, or even that they ought to. Not all citizens are 'experts' and even where they are, this doesn't mean that they can easily navigate the complex situations informed consent as practice places them in. Further, patient expertise/knowledge could be compromised because of the inevitable imbalance of power relations in the clinic setting. This is not to detract from patients' ability to articulate their own knowledge and values claims, but it is important to emphasise that they do so in unequal power conditions.

To identify this range of concerns with informed consent is not to write it off as a framework for negotiating risk, half a loaf presumably being better than none, but to identify ways in which informed consent as a specific bio-ethical and legal framework could be improved, in consultation with the many stakeholders and 'embodied experts' – patients, for example – who navigate informed consent criteria in different contexts. To state that individuals negotiating informed consent can be confused by detail, by the lack of certain types of information, and/or the presenting of information in a certain way, by the setting, by uncertainty, and the difficulties of assessing risk/benefit calculations, is *not* to say that people cannot and should not navigate these decisions, as there is plenty of evidence to suggest that they are able to do so with great skill. But an important issue remains as to what it is they are being informed by, in what circumstances and by whom. It is essential that informed consent, designed as a specific bio-ethical principle and as a legal 'flak jacket' (Herring 2006) for medical practitioners is not seen as the be-all and end-all in terms of debating what is at stake, for individuals, their families, and for society as a whole. In particular, narrow guidelines of informed consent criteria have been argued to 'frame out' broader social and political issues, as here in relation to the HFEA eggs consultation: 'The narrow and specific framing of the consultation questions prevent us from talking about, for example, the wider social context within which women will be expected to make decisions and the inequalities the schemes will exacerbate and produce' (Plows *et al.* 2006: 6).

Section two: choice and choosing: 'individual choice?'

'Individual choice' is perhaps the most commonly heard way in which choice is used in the context of human genetics, and is the focus in this second section. Key issues about choice in the context of human genetics raised by different publics can be summarised as:

- Choices are important for the individual.
- Choices have consequences and carry responsibilities.

Public discourse about human genetics frequently enrols the terms 'individual choice', 'informed choice', 'freedom of choice' and a 'right to choose'.

Discourses which emphasise the primacy of individual rights, autonomy, agency and responsibility have been the primary framing of many of the debates and 'best practice' policy guidelines on genetics. It is important to focus on the voices of patient groups here, many of whom, for example, want access to genetic information and frame this in terms of it being their 'individual choice'. The choice frame is used in a number of very varied circumstances related to human genetics: whether an individual is having a test, undertaking a procedure, having a treatment, or taking a drug. Or, importantly, not having it:

> Some people choose not to have transplants ... Again it's individual choice. You can be a patient and not want treatment. Some people, if they've had ... aggressive treatment for 18 years they will turn around and say well no, I'm not having it any more, I'd rather go, and it's their choice.
>
> ('Susan')

There is a compelling, commonly heard argument for individual choice in many different circumstances, related generally to a narrative of choosing to have, or not to have, something which is offered. 'Susan's' comment below on testing is again a standard discourse:

> it has to be a matter of choice and saying well this is available. It's like genetic testing, I've spoken to lots of people who are anti it, oh, I couldn't have that because I wouldn't really want to know ... but there's going to be another hundred people to that person who say actually, I would like to know.
>
> ('Susan')

Importantly, often the thing which is being offered (the test, the procedure) is seen as neutral. Susan describes it as something which is simply 'available'. The active 'choice' is constructed as being that of the individual. The emphasis on individual 'choice' as a patient-led principle in genetics/reproductive contexts appears in numerous policy documents, such as in HGC and NSC literature. Concepts of individual autonomy, rights and agency enrolled by the discourse of 'individual choice' in a medical setting are hugely important and there is a logic in supporting individual autonomy, especially in relation to what one does with one's own body. Human rights in relation to individual (bodily) autonomy are germane to the debate here. Thus, in exceptionally difficult terrain such as to test or not to test, to tell or not to tell, to take the drug or not, there is a compelling logic to agree with the arguments put forward by the patient groups and other voices who are saying that they are making choices for themselves and that that is up to them.

Individual choice is one of the key frames used by what are termed here 'Libertarian' actors which include the groups the Institute of Ideas, Progress Educational Trust, Sense About Science and also a number of specific 'pro genetics' patient groups such as Genetic Interest Group. The term Libertarian[3] relates to the way in which individual autonomy defined in terms of 'choice' is given value as an ethical, even a political principle. Libertarian 'prime movers' from amongst this network have been extremely visible in many public UK stem cells debates,[4] and also in relation to genetic testing and screening.[5]

As in perhaps no other arena, the framing of choice, especially by these Libertarian prime movers, in relation to genetics and reproduction often sets up an extreme polarisation. Chapter 2 and chapter 5 showed that there is a tendency for very different, complex and ambivalent debates on genetics and reproduction, prenatal screening (PGD, PND), and the use of eggs and embryos for research to be automatically reified and constructed in terms of 'pro life' 'versus' pro choice. We have seen that many are complaining that these either/or framings, common to policy, are not helpful in situations of high complexity, where to voice concerns about 'A' does not necessarily mean one is 'B'. The framing of the debates in terms of (reproductive) 'choice' has meant that to voice concern immediately frames one as anti (reproductive) choice. This has been particularly difficult for feminists and others wishing to raise concerns about PGD or egg donation, because pro-life or anti abortion groups put the status of the embryo first and do not support reproductive choice for women. This conundrum has been addressed by Disability Rights activists (chapter 5).

The issue therefore is whether the framing of the debate in terms of 'choice' is stopping a constructive conversation about the implications of these procedures. An important counter-argument to charges of being 'anti choice' is that these [individual] 'choices' have implications for others and also for the individuals supposedly doing the 'choosing'. Patients also tend to be very aware of the difficulties with 'choice', for instance that choices have consequences and responsibilities, such as who to tell in circumstances of familial genetics testing (chapter 5). 'Sustainability citizenship' prime movers in particular have argued that the discourse of protecting the individual's 'right to choose' can mask the broader social and political context inherent in such 'individual choices'. Chapter 6 discussed the problems with the 'blaming and framing' issues inherent in the individualising of responsibility for one's own health. The flip side of 'individual choice' is 'individual blame' or at the very least, an individualising of responsibility for some exceptionally difficult decisions. Many are questioning whether the use of 'choice' is always an appropriate framing. These issues are developed further in the following subsections which provide situated examples.

The 2006 HFEA consultation *Donating eggs for research: safeguarding donors* represented an important line-drawing moment for many feminists, regarding the use of a discourse of choice by the HFEA in relation to reproductive technologies, and specifically the sourcing and use of women's eggs for cloning purposes, discussed in chapter 2. A workshop to discuss this HFEA consultation took place in November 2006. The workshop concluded that the use of the word 'choice' in the HFEA document implies that to block women from 'choosing' to donate is to deny them individual (reproductive) 'choice'. This inevitably produces an unnecessarily difficult clash between those supportive of 'reproductive choice' as a principle; and those who, while equally supportive of female reproductive autonomy, identify broader issues in the context of such 'choices' accruing to the fallout of global political [bio] economy (Schneider and Schumann 2002; Schneider 2007; Sexton 1999, 2005; Dickenson 2002, 2007). The workshop document produced in response to the HFEA consultation (Plows *et al.* 2006) emphasised the political situated-ness of the issue; even if women are in some cases proactively wishing to 'donate' – or trade – eggs (chapter 2), this is a situation which has been catalysed by the needs of the scientists and also the demands of the 'bio-economy' (chapter 4). In other words, these 'choices' have been set up by specific processes. Further, there was an explicit unpacking of the 'reproductive choice' feminist minefield, as addressed in the workshop document:

> The questionnaire frames the issue of egg donation for research in terms of 'allowing' ... women ... to 'choose' to donate eggs to research: the issue should be framed the other way around in terms of whether researchers should be allowed to approach women ... The issue should not be framed in terms of individual choice, nor should the consultation imply that respondents with concerns about the process of donation are denying women's agency or ability to make choices.
>
> (Plows *et al.* 2006)

Uncoupling a critique of egg donation from the framing of reproductive choice is a significant step which may enable more constructive debates to occur in future, beyond the 'pro or anti choice' framing. Locating individual genetic responsibility for one's health in a social and political landscape (chapter 6), 'sustainability citizenship' prime movers are highlighting the broader social context in which people are making these 'choices' – the political landscape which shapes the individual's 'choice': 'it's a certain understanding of the notion of choice, it ignores the whole structure in which you're presented with all this information in the first place' ('Lucy'). Many say that these are not 'individual choices', so much as individualised decisions which bear heavy burdens of responsibility. Even patient groups who welcome access to genetic tests and prenatal screening are still aware and concerned about the implications and consequences these may have for themselves and others (chapter 5). 'Susan', for example, notes that

> It's great if you find out [that] you're prone to diabetes or something that can be treated, it's going to be hell if you're told that you've got Huntington's or Parkinson's which there's no cure and ... you're predisposed to a condition where there is no hope.
>
> ('Susan')

Writing about her experiences with carrying the breast cancer BRCA1 gene and the pros and cons of testing the younger members of her family for carrier status, Elizabeth Bryan noted that 'being at risk ... is an emotionally ambiguous state ... and could invoke fear, anxiety, envy, hostility or excessive dependency. Imposing upsetting or unwanted information on the younger generation requires careful thought'. (Bryan 2007: 302). The huge weight carried by those facing decisions about whether or not to have a genetic test in specific circumstances was discussed in more detail in chapter 5. 'Choosing' to have a test can have huge consequences and these are highly complex, highly sensitive arenas. Even if one 'chooses' to have a test or undertake a procedure, this does not mean that these 'choices' are easily made; often, quite the reverse. Does a discourse of 'individual choice' allow for a mature debate which captures these complexities? In certain circumstances, affected individuals carry what might be termed a 'burden of choice', and possibly feel a sense of responsibility to 'do the right thing'. Perhaps this is especially the case where genetic screening is offered in an 'opt-out' format, such as PND for Down's syndrome (chapter 5). Many interviewees struggled with trying to reconcile principles of individual autonomy, particularly in relation to reproductive choice, and the consequences of those 'choices'.

> if you know you've got a Down's syndrome child, then once you have that knowledge you're making a choice whether that person comes into existence or not ... you're making choices for that future human being ... I'd probably argue that it's easier to not know.
>
> ('Dave')

Duties, rights and responsibilities (chapter 6) are also inherent in such 'individual choices'. What is expected of the citizen when a specific test is offered in specific circumstances (Plows and Boddington 2006)? Further, in relation to reproduction and genetics, these are 'choices' which produce gendered burdens of responsibility. Several 'sustainability citizenship' interviewees had a very dystopian diagnosis of future UK health policy in relation to how genetics information is increasingly being used in tandem with reproductive technologies, forecasting that PND could be used as a means of forcing people to abort foetuses with genetic conditions as a cost saving to the NHS.

> the NHS is being privatised by the back door ... within the area of pregnancy, if the [prenatal genetic] test says your child is likely to have this disability, and we won't give you health care ... what choice is that for a woman in a society that is very individualistic and does not give help?
>
> ('Lucy')

'Lucy' is predicting that healthcare provision in the future could be withdrawn from people who might decide to keep a disabled baby, or even perhaps a baby diagnosed as 'predisposed' to develop a genetic condition. This may seem like extreme paranoia. However, the debates on the 'right to die' (triggered again in October 2008 through the death of a 23-year-old in the Swiss clinic 'Dignitas' (*The Guardian* 2008c)) and concerns about this 'right' becoming framed as a 'duty' are very relevant to debates on 'choice' and consent within human genetics. Many have spoken on how voluntary euthanasia could easily become a co-opted concept, with old people becoming pressured in various ways – even unintentionally – into seeing themselves as a burden and 'choosing' euthanasia.

Market discourse and practice has a bearing on 'choice', not least because the word 'choice' is often linked in different contexts to the term 'consumer choice'. An analysis of the 'bio-economy' (chapter 4) makes an important contribution to the broader framing of background conditions which set up these so-called 'individual choices'. There is a global need for 'bio-resources', which is an identifiable driver of what creates specific 'individual choices'. Bio-economic discourses and practices set up the 'bio-sphere' as a resource to be mined, through the production and use of bio-material which has 'bio-value' (Waldby 2002). These demands of the bio-economy drive the creation of specific situations which are subsequently framed in terms of individual choice and consent in specific contexts. Examples include the 'trade' (Dickenson 2007) in human eggs from Eastern Europe and India to the West (chapter 2), and the political economy of 'choosing' – for example, to be a drugs trial subject or to donate bio-material – when there is a financial or other incentive. How well are risks weighed by those participating out of financial or other need, such as wishing to have IVF? Chapter 5 gave the example of how genetic tests are being marketed as products, sold on the open market to the public-as-bio-consumer, exercising market 'freedom of choice' through buying commercially available tests which often have questionable medical value; but have very real financial value to the sellers.

Another problem with 'choosing' is that choices hold implicit and/or explicit value(s), and this is extremely difficult for the people faced with making them, not least because there are many different ways of valuing and they are not mutually exclusive. The values we place on different human traits are another way of understanding the concept of 'bio-value' (Waldby 2002). Again, genetics and reproduction is a hotly debated arena in relation to a range of increasingly available 'choices' which carry values. Information cannot be seen as simply neutral but is valued in various ways, depends on a person's values and the associated meanings they give to the information. Chapter 5 provides examples of how different individuals have different assessments and responses to the same disease conditions. There are values, for instance, accruing to screening out embryos carrying specific traits such as Down's syndrome or Cystic Fibrosis through PND and PGD (chapter 5). People want 'normal', 'healthy' babies and many talk of a 'right to choose' to have a 'normal' baby. This sounds fair enough, but what does 'normal' imply? Where would society draw the line? In fact the line is shifting rapidly as the range of available tests broadens. Choices and values can imply discrimination and stigma – that 'this is ok, but this isn't'. Is it possible to choose to screen out conditions such as Down's without placing negative value on lives of those living with them? These issues place the people tasked with making these sorts of 'choices' in a very difficult position.

The Disability Rights groups and other 'sustainability citizenship' actors who are voicing concern about PGD and PND and in some cases calling this a eugenics policy, are careful to say that they do not wish to point the finger at specific individuals such as those with carrier status for 'serious' heritable genetic conditions who are in the front line of bearing the burden of having to 'choose' value-laden options. Rather, they aim to locate these choices, saying that it is vital to think about ways to have a broader debate about what we value as a society, and the significance of providing prenatal tests for conditions with no known cures. How do we come to have the attitudes we do towards the things we want to 'screen out'? 'We don't want to judge women who have PND ... [these are] difficult decisions ... the question is who is making the decision and how is it being made?' (European feminist campaign network 'ReproKult' member, ESF workshop, London 2004). And also, why is it being made. The issue of sex selection of embryos for so-called 'social' reasons is a clear example of values-laden 'choices'.

While some critique the use of PND and PGD in terms of the implicit values they see being placed on children, others will view the possibility of choosing for, or choosing to screen out, different characteristics in a positive way, enrolling alternative value frameworks. A woman carrying the BRCA1 breast cancer gene may well wish to have PGD in order to ensure that any daughter she has is born free of the condition, because the value she places on the life of her future baby means that she does not want her baby to live under the threat of developing cancer. In 2009 the first baby selected via PGD to be free of the BRCA1 gene was born, sparking a debate in the media about where society would draw the line in relation to selecting embryos free of specific genes which may, but also may not, cause specific diseases (*The Guardian* 2009a). This has been the subject of debate on breast cancer chat boards (Macmillan 2009). It is precisely because these issues are so complex and difficult that they have been framed in terms of choice, leaving it up to the individual to choose. But to reiterate an important point, this places a burden of choice on the individual, and these tests have been socially, politically and economically produced – they did not just suddenly become 'available'.

Choosing *for* – positive choice and trait selection – has also become possible, through the 'saviour siblings' test case which was allowed by the Court of Appeal in 2003 (HFEA 2003) (chapter 5). Again such 'choices' are value-laden, in a variety of ways. Particularly in relation to the 'saviour siblings' example, Human Genetics Alert (HGA) has voiced strong concerns about commodification and market-led values in relation to 'choosing' characteristics of children through PGD/IVF. HGA sees this as the thin end of the wedge, prefigurative of social moves towards 'designer babies' through choosing for or screening out genetic traits in specific embryos:

> Social prejudices and market forces could create a 'positive' eugenics in which parents selected the 'best' from amongst multiple embryos, based upon their own choice of both health and non-health-related criteria (such as sex, appearance, aptitudes etc.).

> (HGA 2000)

At an 'ethics café' meeting in London, in June 2003, a participant framed the choosing of a saviour sibling in terms of commodification. Were the parents having a baby – or 'having a factory for bone marrow?'.[5] The concern about the values implications of 'choosing for' framed in terms of commodification and 'designer babies' is quite prevalent amongst objections from 'members of the public' (chapters 5 and 8).

Conclusion: broadening the frame

The protection of the individual in medical settings has been developed against background histories of appalling experimentation including Nazi research and eugenics programmes (Kerr and Shakespeare 2002). Human rights legislation has been developed specifically to protect individual rights. There are thus important reasons why the terms and concepts of consent and choice are now prevalent in UK legislature and public and policy discourse. This chapter however has identified some key problems with choice and consent, in particular how these terms are framing debates along certain lines, which can be misleading and lead to skewed debates which 'frame out' other important perspectives or mean that they are not easily heard. It is important to set the debates on some different tracks; to broaden, or to tilt, the frame.

Policy makers can be seen to make assumptions about the best way to conduct the debates and what issues are at stake. The critiques of informed consent and informed choice summarised in this chapter have shown where some of the holes in policy-led accounts are. Informed consent, informed choice and individual choice, to reiterate, are often not up to the task and are heavily laden with subliminal meanings. These are not 'value-neutral' concepts. In relation to informed consent or informed choice, it is pertinent to ask: Informed by what? By whom? In what context? Attention has tended to focus on the words choice and consent, but it is also important to critically examine the term 'informed' which often accompanies them, as the 2006 feminist workshop on HFEA egg sourcing did. Many are saying that we need to talk more about the broader social context, about power relations, and values, where we as a society want to be. In essence, this situates debates about genetics firmly within debates about citizenship and citizenship stakes, and this would appear to encourage a broader and less polarised discussion. It is important to have a debate which identifies the responsibilities and duties which accrue in relation to human genetics, and how these are unevenly spread. The ReproKult spokeswoman quoted earlier used the word *decision*, rather than choice. Would it help to talk about informed decisions rather than individual choices (Schmitz *et al.* 2009)?

The chapter has provided specific examples of the limits or problems with the use of choice and consent to frame the debates. When developed for a specific medical practice, informed consent is arguably based on limited criteria which fail to provide the 'bigger picture' necessary to make the right decision. Informed consent, arguably, is an ethical and legal 'flak jacket' (Herring 2006) for the practitioner; while it may be 'good enough' (Corrigan 2003) for legal cover, it can be seen in specific cases such as the procurement of eggs or DNA samples to be inadequate to the task at hand. 'Choice' is in danger of becoming a reified moral stand-in for a range of other ethical principles and values, especially in terms of the values people place on life, their own identity and health, and the lives of others. It is difficult to hear, above the 'freedom of choice' and 'right to individual choice' discourses in the context of genetics, the voices of those who wish to talk about concepts of value and worth, of threats to their own identity and very existence through screening programmes, and above all to locate politically the discourse of choice. Many groups and individuals, including the patient group 'prime movers' who generally support genetics research and applications, explicitly articulate complexity and ambivalence when they discuss 'choice', particularly in relation to genetic testing and screening. These are massively sensitive and difficult arenas, as they cut to the heart of many of the health and identity debates and frames articulated by key actor groups and perhaps Disability Rights and patient groups in particular. Because these issues deal with real people and their lives, extreme caution needs to be used, in terms of conducting a balanced, fair, politically aware and constructive debate on human genetics either over general principles or in terms of specific case examples.

There are no easy answers to the ethical conundrums set in motion by the increasing use of genetic and associated technologies in everyday life, but we can at least construct more sensitive means of conducting the debates, and better forms of participatory democracy. It is essential to break out of the debate framed in terms of people being 'for or anti' individual choice or informed consent in specific contexts, as this sets people against each other and polarises the debate in unhelpful ways. Critics of genetic tests, and the patient groups who might wish to have them, have plenty to say to each other beyond such tired discussions.

We now turn in the final chapter to examine the different forms of 'futures talk' which are often used by different publics in relation to specific aspects and implications of human genetics.

8 Futures talk

Introduction

The invocation of the future permeates genetics/genomics discourse; key futures talk can be summarised as 'future promise' (Brown and Michael 2003) and 'future risk'. Importantly, both are contested future territory; what counts as a risk, or a benefit? Benefits; progress; risk; hope; hype; predictability; uncertainty; 'futures trading'; 'future good' (altruism on behalf of future generations), are all important forms of futures talk, discussed in this chapter. The invoked future in genetics discourse is based on a projection of the present, based both on the values people (and groups, institutions, cultures, societies) hold, and their socio-political and economic predictions, assessments and imperatives about where 'the science' will, might or should go. Thus future predictions are based on competing accounts of current worldviews, and can be seen as a means of persuasion about why specific courses of action should or shouldn't be followed. This idea of the future, multiple futures, based on fluid, subjective accounts of the present, shaped by political, social and economic forces, has been recently raised in relation to nanotechnology (Nordmann 2008). Throughout the book, we have seen how specific groups – especially amongst 'sustainability citizenship' networks – have critiqued the power relations and vested interests which enable others to have more influence in setting the stakes of the debate; and hence to colonise the future with a specific account. For example, chapter 4 and chapter 5 identified links between the demands of the 'bio-economy' and 'future promise' discourse about what the scientific and economic benefits will be, as framed by specific actor groups; a form of 'futures trading'.

Certain discourses with a very powerful resonance such as a patient's hopes for a cure, or promissory discourse on personalised pharmaco are thus staking strong claims on the future. This puts groups with less public visibility and power, or those whose frames have less immediate 'purchase', at a disadvantage, as they are not able to frame their own visions of the future on their own terms, but only in relation to the future framing of others; a key complaint raised repeatedly in relation to policy consultations, as we have seen. Certain groups, wary of the ways and means by which genetic science is being introduced into society, are more predisposed to identify risks and grievances arising from the way the future is being framed by others or implicit in these accounts and procedures. Such risk framings are generally based on past experience, for example of environmental controversies (Nelkin 1995; Plows and Reinsborough 2008), which tend to be heard less over 'future promise' accounts, even though risk management is a key regulatory principle. However prime movers are also resisting this reactive risk framing, wanting instead to focus on what they are *for*; to put forward their own 'future promise' accounts. It is, however, harder to get these essentially non-genetic discourses (such as poverty alleviation) framed in what can be extremely geneticised debates, for example, in terms of how future generations will be healthy (chapter 6).

Futures discourse, especially future promise, has profound implications for policy; how health budgets are spent, for example. Genetic 'progress' (advances, benefits) is defined in terms of maximising health: but the definition of health and routes to achieve it are complex territory (chapter 6). Future accounts of genetics are of particular relevance in terms of the impacts they are having on, for example:

- health policy
- social policy
- economics: futures trading, investment
- law – (for example, the HFEA Act 2008)
- reflection of cultural values – what counts as 'progress'.

Specific groups tend to be repeatedly named as future beneficiaries, or framed as at future risk; for example children, future generations, specific disease communities, patient groups, the disabled, the poor, women. A familiar list of cures and treatments and disease prevention is enrolled in promissory accounts relating to a variety of techniques and applications, whether stem cells or pharmacogenomics. Much of the promise is medical promise: we will get new treatments, we will get cures, we will improve existing treatments. Cures may be further away than treatments which merely alleviate conditions, but in the meantime, we can be kept going on the allure of 'hope'. The promise of genetics exists for current individuals, and also for future generations, and claims accruing to such 'future altruism' accompany many calls for public support in the here and now of medical research of various types, including the donation of bio-material; as we have seen, often a contested issue, which tends to rely heavily on accounts of 'future promise' to persuade present day publics to participate (chapter 3).

Competing accounts of future promise and future risk, to reiterate, importantly enrol a debate about norms and values. Utopias and dystopias invoke an imagined future, which can get people stuck in a debate about what is or is not scientifically viable; but essentially the debate is really about what values are at stake in the here and now: one person's utopia is another's dystopia. It is not just that the scientific and technological basis of many claims can often be problematic; the underlying values shaping such claims also need scrutiny. Genetics brings not only a medical promise, but the possibility of enhancing our species, and with it the potential that future generations may transcend mere humanity: the transhuman or the superhuman may lie ahead. We are potentially building a new world of humans free of certain diseases, a world of possible life extension. But whose future is this? Who wants what? Is enhancement 'progress'? and what actually constitutes 'better' humans? (Wilsden and Miller 2006). Habermas is preoccupied with 'the future of human nature', locating his concerns in an economic account of 'market-led eugenics' (Habermas 2003). Fukuyama (2002), however, is excited by the potential for 'our posthuman future'.

Transhumanism and life extension are very much discourses of the rich West, while much of the world dies young through poverty and easily pre-ventable diseases which do not require high-tech genomic fixes. Such future promise thus invokes a hornet's nest of contested norms and values. We need to think clearly about who will benefit, and in what ways, from any deliveries on the future promise of genetics, and compare the promises being made about genetics with the critiques that it will exacerbate social injustice. There may be progress in cures, in treatments which might not be cures as such, but which might lead to amelioration of medical problems; progress in diag-nosis, which might or might not lead to cures or other treatments. However there are problems with straightforwardly seeing all these goals as progress or benefits; these are contested terms. Not everyone will have the same atti-tude towards prenatal testing and selective implantation or abortion, for exam-ple. From a scientific and technical viewpoint, it might be straightforward to see the development of screening tests for various genetic conditions as 'pro-gress' – we can do something we could not do before. But, if there are no cures or treatments for these conditions, the practice of implementing these tests presents, for affected individuals, families and communities, arguably, meagre progress, or even a positive burden (chapter 5). As we have seen, the provision of extra choices does not straightforwardly and in all cases count as a benefit.

The following sections give examples of typical ways in which the future is invoked, identifying different types of futures talk such as invocations of pre-dictability, or when hope blurs to hype. The chapter identifies in what con-texts such futures talk manifests itself and how different publics invoke or respond to these frames. We begin with a short examination of 'time talk' more generally in genetics discourse.

The past and present are often invoked or implied in genetics discourse; for example, the white paper *Our inheritance, our future* (Dept of Health 2003) clearly uses concepts of the past to invoke the future. The past is mobilised in genetics discourse, usually in terms of DNA, heritability, identity and 'belonging'. The quest for origins, and for meaning, is something humans like to do; telling stories of 'belonging' to different communities, families. Genetic information is being used in a number of interdisciplinary studies to trace demographic geographical patterns and spread over time. Popular television programmes have used reality TV formats, for example to trace Viking ancestry and patterns through DNA. Off the back of its own privately funded human DNA database, National Geographic have started running luxury tours consisting of visits to far-flung indigenous tribal groups whose DNA is part of the composite 'human genome'. All these practices, using genetics to construct meanings about the past, origins, identity and belonging, link to the geneticisation discussions in chapter 6. Tests on present family members – genetic testing for heritable familial conditions – also invoke a 'looking back' to previous generations and family history. The past, heritability, is thus enrolled to construct meanings about the future; the implications of the inherited genetic information for specific individuals, and the decisions – 'choices' – they might make (chapter 5).

The past is also invoked in terms of 'lessons for the future'-style narratives, perhaps most often in terms of warnings: for example eugenics 'lessons from the past', or comparisons with nuclear energy and genetics, interestingly often in relation to the hyping of future benefits and underplaying of risk. This is made explicit in the title of a recent book chapter: 'Technological Challenges: Asbestos Past Experiences, Nanoparticles Future Developments' (Rahman 2008). And in an interview with a technology watchdog campaigner:

> I went to an event at the Royal Society in London on gene therapy, about 1992, 1994 ... And it was all tremendously positive. But ... having been in the nuclear industry I'm thinking, we've heard all this before.
>
> ('James')

What is very noticeable about the present in much genetics discourse from specific groups, is how it is framed as the almost-future by the discourse of society being on the brink of scientific 'breakthroughs', where speed is of the essence: 'it's ... snowballed really ... it shows how quickly science is moving and how quickly new research is coming on board, thank god ... some people have died waiting for it and we've got kids that need it now' ('Susan'). 'Nanoscience and nanotechnologies are evolving rapidly, and the pressures of international competition will ensure that this will continue' (Royal Society 2004). There is a kind of 'Alice in Wonderland' white rabbit-ness about such talk – must rush, can't stop, no time. The present moment is almost always associated with speed, with pushing forward, with an accompanying ethical imperative; people need treatments now; they are 'just around the corner' (Evans *et al.* 2008). Risk assessment procedures are often framed as 'unethical' by various 'pro science' lobby groups because they 'slow down' research. Time, speed and research future outcomes are thus invariably linked in accounts of where the science is at in the here and now. The bio-economy and industry links to the present-as-almost-future trope are important too; competitiveness itself as a discourse also invokes the present in terms of the future – being 'ahead in the race' to stake out territory in the bio-economy, in the knowledge economy.

The remainder of this chapter is divided into sections which each address a specific type, or set of types, of 'futures talk'.

Prediction and uncertainty

Prediction and uncertainty in relation to human genetics invoke the future; this both emerges from, and has consequences for, the present moment, in ways which are summarised below through selected examples. In chapter 6, genetic determinism was seen to stake out a genetic 'future heritage' as being something unchangeable. The medical and scientific reality is that our genetic future heritage is more mutable and uncertain.

Prediction, especially in relation to genetic/genomic predisposition and susceptibility to disease, invokes, indeed forecasts, the future. The scientific viability of predictive testing is very context-dependent, ranging from certainty relating to disease expression, to extreme uncertainty (chapters 3, 6). Genetic/ genomic prediction invokes and potentially creates a specific account of the future. It potentially privileges a geneticised account of health, invokes contested outcomes and values, and catalyses accounts of social and environmental justice goals in relation to health (chapter 6). The limits of prediction have been a recurring theme, for example chapter 3 identified that predicting disease expression on the basis of information about a 'single-gene disorder' is different to modelling predictions for broad populations' susceptibility to common complex diseases. There are thus competing accounts and confusion over what the future may hold: 'I don't think we are going to have everything predicted from our genome' ('Jenny'). The social justice implications of genetic/ genomic predictability (putting its scientific viability to one side) are considerable, but can be summarised by the potential for individualised responsibility to 'blame and frame' groups and individuals and ignore the social context; for example, the causes of pollution, or the existence of poverty (chapter 6).

Predictive testing for susceptibility across a spectrum raises many ethical concerns. A key issue is how individuals may react to the information in terms of an imagined future:

> predictive medicine ... implies something about the future, that you may carry this gene and this gives you a susceptibility to something ... how far should you go in telling people information that may just be simply giving them more to worry about? ... it's not an automatic presumption that genetic knowledge is necessarily a good thing.
>
> ('James')

Chapter 5 provides examples on how the use of predictive genetic testing at prenatal level catalyses highly sensitive ethical debates about preventing the existence of babies which would otherwise be born with specific conditions.

Uncertain economic and political futures affect scientific uncertainty as well as the viability and replicability of the science itself. Reflecting this, much 'future promise' genetics/genomics discourse actually has many ifs and buts and hopefullys built into promissory accounts of cures and treatments for disease (in particular). There is also a standard phrase, 'in five to ten years' which accompanies much discourse about the translation of medical 'breakthroughs' into viable applications:

> gene therapy in CF wasn't a huge success in the beginning but it now looks as if it's moving in that direction ... When we got involved in '92, Bob Williamson was talking about it being ... five to ten years down the line, we're now twelve years down the line.
>
> ('Susan')

> it may be decades before any result comes through
>
> ('Peter')

This caution interestingly co-exists with speed and 'rapid progress' talk, all from the same sorts of groups: scientists, regulators, patients and lobby groups, reiterating that a recurring theme of genetic promise is that of speed, often coupled with urgency. Uncertain futures thus co-exist with discourses that change is projected to happen in the very near future, and the necessity of this. Discussing medical/scientific uncertainty, some draw analogies with other unfulfilled promises of scientific hype: 'Xenotransplantation was going to be the big thing five years ago and now hardly anyone is talking about it so there's huge ... uncertainty in all this' ('Peter'). From 'Peter', a medical charity spokesperson, this talk is first of all reasonable and responsible caution, given the scientific uncertainties identified not just by various watchdogs, but also by himself and many others within medical and scientific networks. It is also partly self-interest around keeping funders, and 'the general public' on board, and hence being wary of hype. 'Susan', a pro research patient spokesperson, is keen to emphasise the need to keep on with research despite such uncertainty:

> When Christian Barnard did the first heart transplant, it wasn't quite what they were expecting, but they didn't stop. I think that's the important thing of any technology ... research is not 100 per cent perfect, that's why it's called research.
>
> ('Susan')

This invokes a faith in future outcomes; hope for the future of a specific, familiar type; cures and treatments.

Risk

Defining risks, and the focus on risks rather than benefits, is a debate in the present moment which relates to contested views of the future; a debate in which some have more legitimacy than others. Risk is a key way the future is constructed and enrolled in genetics discourse; different actors aim to forecast the future through identifying potential future risks, sometimes referred to in policy contexts as 'horizon scanning' (Defra 2002). Many watchdogs focus their attention on horizon scanning for future risks: 'we ... spend a lot of time with scientific technologists engaging with them, usually on future issues. We have a particular aim of trying to find the issues that are going to be the ... forthcoming ones' ('James'). Risk is a core concept in relation to public attitudes to, and governance of, human genetics, influenced in part by Ulrich Beck's definition of a contemporary 'risk society' (Beck 1992, 1995), predisposed to identify environmental risks, for example. Governance is especially concerned with ensuring safety through identifying risks, and in certain contexts such as human clinical trials for drugs, there are extremely detailed criteria for identifying risks. In specific circumstances, risk management is very effective, and there are a plethora of guidelines for identified risk avoidance, safety protocols, best practice, ethical codes of conduct, relating to different R&D procedures.

Risk management as policy can be characterised as an aim to achieve a balance between groups who identify risks and uncertainties and the different stakeholders (patients, scientists, commercial interests) pushing research forward. It is debatable how much of a balance actually exists, however. Some very worrying policy gaps exist in relation to risks even when these are basic safety ones – for example, ETC states that only a 'handful' of toxicology studies on nanotech exist, even though there are hundreds of nano-products already on the market (Plows and Reinsborough 2008). Risk governance in policy generally is about weighing (known, likely, potential) risks and (known, likely, potential) benefits, in Europe informed by the 'Precautionary Principle' (Jasanoff 1995; Ahteensuu 2004; Horlick Jones, Walls, Rowe, *et al.* 2007; Salter and Jones 2002). The precautionary principle, in essence, states that if there is a chance of catastrophic ill results, risks should not be taken even for the sake of possibly large gain. Critics argue that a very 'weak' version of the Precautionary Principle in fact operates, even in the EU, which has a much 'tougher' approach to issues of risk than the USA, for example. A very 'strong' version of the Precautionary Principle would of course mean that no research would be carried out at all; it being impossible to prove unquantifiable, uncertain or unknown risks by their very nature. This very uncertainty is also a form of risk, in fact a core mobilising frame for many actors who say that genetics applications will produce unquantifiable outcomes in 'the lab without walls' (Szerszynski 2005).

UK/EU policy-led risk management is thus arguably more about the management of public concerns about risk, rather than managing the risks themselves. Tellingly, an aim of public engagement (chapter 1) is to win 'public confidence' via the policy process through clear 'risk management'. There are economic considerations at stake: 'Without broad public acceptance and support, the development and use of life sciences and biotechnology in Europe will be contentious, benefits will be delayed and competitiveness will be likely to suffer' (CEC 2002: 19). The importance of the bio-economy to nation states is considerable (chapter 4), to the point where economic concerns clearly outweigh other considerations.

Risk assessment as policy involves important debates in terms of what counts as a risk and who gets to define this. This is stake-setting, which not only produces an account of the future, but in very significant ways actually brings this future into being through what is allowed and what is not. Tellingly, civil society actors who frame risks rather than benefits tend to have fewer 'strong ties' links with governance and powerful elites; they thus have less influence in staking out the future, and strenuously campaign about this imbalance in power relations, generally citing the power and influence which bio-industry such as 'big pharma' exerts in this domain (ETC 2008b, Birch 2006). Importantly, risks relate to worldviews; what gets defined as a risk by policy/governance is generally narrower than what counts as a risk for civil society:

> studies on risk perception indicate that lay people perceive risks differently from scientific experts ... Experts tend to keep the problem within what they perceive to be a purely technical frame, whereas lay people implicitly emphasise behavioural, cultural, social and economic aspects.
>
> (Torgersen *et al.* 2003: 75)

As part of efforts to ensure 'upstream' public engagement, risk identification can in theory be given quite full scope; however policy is generally made solely on the assessment of scientific criteria, itself often very narrowly framed (Horlick-Jones, Walls, Kitzinger *et al.* 2007). This is frustrating for many participants wishing to frame the debate along broader lines. Hence, grievances with policy process relating to how risks are identified and governed are core reasons why publics mobilise in opposition. Public engagement, power and policy processes – how stakes are set – are thus core to campaign groups' risk framing; this is as much about the here and now, as it is about the future. Groups identifying broader, or less accepted, types of risks are doing well to get them identified as such at all, especially given that many groups struggle to have 'stakeholder' status in the first place and that the public arguably still suffers from a 'deficit model' hangover.

A further concern for groups who are predisposed to identify risks, is how risk assessment potentially 'buys into' hype:

> you can contribute to the hype in some ways with these technologies ... I feel wary that I might accidentally promote a kind of ... discourse about, 'well, we hear about these amazing miracles but we've got to have the safeguards'. In some cases, that can be true, with some aspects of DNA. In other cases, it's not.
>
> ('Jenny')

This is an important concern about responding to an account of the future which is itself disputed; that getting too locked into discussing risks in terms of where the technology might go, actually helps the process of 'performing the science into being', lending it credence. This is something of a catch-22 situation.

While certain groups struggle to get risks heard and identified in the regulatory sphere, still less have anything done about them, they have other problems too. 'Future benefit' frames relating to treatments and cures trump risk frames on many levels, not least in terms of the emotional claims staked out by, or on behalf of, future beneficiaries. The imperative for cures is often used as an argument to overcome any other considerations, such as research involving animals or human embryos. Risk as an invocation of the future simply loses out to such emotive 'future promise': 'Clearly the rights crowd who are so against this don't have any members suffering terminal illness that could be cured by such experimentation' (Email on chat list personally accessed by the author, 2005); 'some people have died waiting for [research results] and we've got kids now that need it now. I wish someone could take [Animal Rights activists] to a hospital and they can see children lying there dying of cancers' ('Susan'). Many in fact say that that risk governance simply gets in the way of finding cures. A genetics statistician, speaking during the Institute of Ideas' 'Genes and Society' event in 2003, said that 'ethical committees are meddling in individual choice'[1] and this is a common frame.

Risk is often defined by certain groups as fear, generally fear of an unknown future;

> 'I do find it very wearying when people [say] "oh science is frightening". Yes, the unknown is frightening, that's the point of research, that you then find out what is unknown or you develop something that is there to benefit people'
>
> ('Susan').

Susan's statement is very typical. Risk, from such a perspective, is seen as something irrational. Libertarian lobby groups such as 'prime movers' the Institute of Ideas (see also Furedi 2002) are very adept at equating risk with fear, saying that publics and campaign groups voice concerns out of fear and ignorance, obstructing patients' legitimate hopes of cures and treatments. Genetic watchdogs such as GeneWatch who identify risks are thus framed as mobilising over irrational fears, while patients who need cures suffer. This is what might be called the 'deficit model' hangover. While there is certainly something to be said for the way 'moral panics' can get triggered, for example in the media (Haran *et al.* 2007), this is not the same as raising concerns about future health risk or querying scientific viability, as genetic watchdogs do. In fact, fear of the future permeates discourse around disease cure and prevention, as 'Lucy' identifies: 'It ... seems that everybody and anybody is prepared to allow ... anything if it's a promise of, 'I will cure you of sickness'. It builds on a fear of death, a fear of being sick and of not being supported' ('Lucy'). 'Lucy' identifies that fear – of becoming ill, of death – can also act to mobilise people in support of genetics research. This contributes to the already powerful emotive argument that 'anything goes' in the name of medical research future promise.

Previous chapters have given situated examples of health and environmental risks. There is much uncertainty about what risks may actually transpire from human genetics applications, especially given the highly experimental stage of the technology. An example of a specific health risk is seen in the high profile death of Jesse Gelsinger, who died following gene therapy in the USA when his body had a massive auto-immune response to the viral vector carrying the gene (Gelsinger 2008); this essentially halted gene therapy trials. The technology watchdog Institute of Science in Society (ISIS) has focused much attention on the potential for bio-engineered viruses associated with techniques such as gene therapy not only to adversely affect the individual, but to create much more widespread health and environmental hazards. Indeed, ISIS warns that novel viral strains may already have entered environmental systems, with impacts on human health: 'SARS virus genetically engineered?' (Ho 2003). Several viral vectors genetically engineered to facilitate uptake of genes into the body in 'cut and paste' gene therapy have been derived from some of the most virulent viruses on the planet, including the cauliflower mosaic virus (Cummins ca. 2008). Concerns about how these might impact on the environment/population health, through accidental release or even as an unintended consequence of a medical procedure, are raised by scientists such as 'Alice' as well as by genetic and technology watchdog and campaign groups.

> viruses being used to introduce gene therapy is very worrying ... potentially a ... huge health hazard. ... new organisms, the new viruses just getting out there and causing who knows what kind of problems ... through the gene therapy patients going out and passing their virus out to people in the street ... no-one's really looking for it are they? So you've just got no way of knowing if it's happening.
>
> ('Alice')

'Alice's' comment that 'no one is looking for it' is significant: if risks are not quantified properly, which they cannot be given the uncertainty of how such technologies will impact with human and eco systems, then there may well be impacts which are not linked to causes; this is ISIS's point in relation to SARS. Another example of an identified health risk is ovarian hyperstimulation (chapter 2).

Significantly, certain groups may choose to discount risks to the point of taking them themselves, such as patients:

> it's like the first AIDS patients who took AZT ... they said ... we'll be the human guinea pigs because we're dying anyway ... and 'Emily' [CF sufferer] did that when she did a drug trial for the Brompton for

the liver because when you know that there isn't anything else, well it might work.

('Susan')

'Emily' made a risk/benefit calculation that this action was worth the risk; a very poignant gamble on future outcomes with highly personal consequences for herself.

'Future promise'

All medical research inherently looks to the future, but genetic research is especially imbued with talk about great 'future promise'. It is a discourse reproduced not only by the patient groups and their advocates, but by those directly involved in the science and associated industrial and commercial activity. It is the key frame on the websites and literature of medical research funders such as Wellcome; and on the websites and literature of the bodies involved in the regulation and governance of the science and technology. There are many associated sorts of future promise including hype and hope and these are differentiated in this section. The book has identified that this 'future promise' relates primarily to the cure, treatment and prevention of specific diseases; a list of 'usual suspects' which appear time and again in different accounts of different technological processes and potential applications. Many are motivated by the desire to contribute to the 'public good' through eradicating disease, not least the scientists:

the enthusiasm [about] the potential of what ... this discovery could do ... and often I think a very altruistic [motivation] ... people genuinely want to make a difference so they fall into that area of science because they want to help people.

('James')

Regulatory examples of 'future promise' discourse include:

Advances in human genetics are being made at a rapid rate. In response to this, the Government needs to: ... ensure an effective strategic advisory and regulatory structure that identifies and maximises benefits from potential advances in human genetics ...

(HGC website 2005)[2]

The very title of the white paper on genetics *Our inheritance, our future* (Dept of Health 2003) highlights this 'future promise' invoked by health policy makers. The World Health Organisation (WHO) identifies future promise but also critiques hype:

An over-optimistic picture of the applications and benefits of genetic research has been drawn. The potential medical applications of genomics are considerable and will lead to major advances in clinical practice but the time-scale is difficult to predict ... It is likely that within the next few years, new diagnostic agents, vaccines and therapeutic agents for communicable diseases will be available. In the same time frame, however, breakthroughs in the diagnosis and management of cancer and new treatments for chronic diseases are far less certain.

(WHO 2005)

Much patient discourse is of hope relating to such 'future promise', for example Seriously Ill for Medical Research (SIMR):

SIMR believes it would be unethical and immoral not to use powerful modern techniques to research the 5,000 single gene disorders which affect 2.5 million people or the major diseases which have a genetic factor, like heart disease, cancer, asthma, diabetes or Alzheimer's disease. Modern biotechnology ... can now offer real hope for conquering many previously incurable illnesses.

(SIMR 2005)

Hope is inherent in much future promise discourse, and is particularly prevalent in patients' narratives, with the urgency of this imperative underlined by medical conditions with a genetic basis which lead to death.

And that's what you're living on, it's a hope ... for some people that's all they've got ... our members ... are looking forward to the future, because so many people are reliant on technology for a better quality of life and for longer lives ... Cures are the gold at the end of the rainbow.

('Susan')

It can be seen how such discourse enrols specific others as future beneficiaries, of which a common example is the very ill child. This is one of the lowest common denominators of medical ethics, known in its more abstract form as the 'desperate case', whose only chance is gene therapy, or stem cell research, or a saviour sibling, or whatever the specific technology, medical research is at stake in this specific case:

It astounds me how people would be happy to see a child die, or suffer severely, when something could be done to save them. I think I'd be very happy to know I'd helped save my sibling's life when I was born.

(Participant on 'saviour siblings' online debate, BBC 2004b)

A sick child is used in an appeal for fund raising and to legislators and policy makers, as well as to those who set priorities for medical research and budgeting. Such discourse features prominently in debate about the direction of future medical research, especially genetic research. Hope for a child's future is at once hope for the future promise of this research. This focuses on the personal, and on the particular case, '[E]very time there's a big new story about research, ... the first thing the media want are the patients, because ... it's human interest ... you want somebody with a face, or a child and that brings the story home' ('Susan'). The undeniable power of the argument resides in various features. A personal case makes vivid the human costs of adhering to certain principles or limits. There comes a point at which most of us would bend any principles by which we live. The focus on a child, an 'innocent' who had nothing to do with creating the ethical rules of engagement, yet stands to lose out because of them, provides the sharpest challenge to those rules. In its reproductive form, this is a future, hoped for child, or an existing healthy child who would not have been born but for new medical or reproductive technologies which may be under technical or ethical challenge. Countering this very emotive use of a single case, a specific child, is exceptionally hard. Anyone countering these arguments head on with a renewed insistence on sticking to principle is likely to be thought very hard-hearted. Hence such a position is rarely adopted publicly or directly: 'You do always have to think about what do I say to the person with the dying child ... ' ('Alice').

A specific form of 'future promise' explicitly enrols future generations as beneficiaries. Future-orientated altruistic discourse is heard from various key sources; from the regulators:

> We all share the same basic human genome ... This sharing of our genetic constitution not only gives rise to opportunities to help others but it also highlights our common interests in the fruits of medically-based genetic research.
>
> (HGC 2002)

Such calls on genetic solidarity and gifting the future especially relate to the UK Biobank's calls to donate DNA samples (chapter 3): 'Taking part is not intended to help you directly but, it should give future generations a much better chance of living their lives free of diseases that disable and kill' (UK Biobank 2008). Much talk from patients is altruistically focused into the future: '"Dave" knew that any research wasn't actually going to help him, but his ambition was that new research and technology would help people coming along behind him who have been diagnosed with the condition' ('Susan').

However, benefits are contested territory; appeals to 'future altruism' around donation of bio-material have raised concerns, for example, in relation to eggs (chapter 2) and DNA samples (chapter 3). Does 'anything go'? 'If through human engineering we can bring an end to human suffering ... we have an obligation to many future lives that have yet to be lived' (Email on chat list accessed by the author, 2005).

Hype is another specific type of future promise talk. Critiques of hype come from a range of sources, not to mention those involved in the science who critique others' use of it. It has been suggested that there was a great deal of genetic hype, associated with the millennium, but that it is now much more tempered, with the exception of certain avid enthusiasts, particularly in relation to 'futures trading'. This itself has caused a backlash, especially in relation to gene therapy, which had very much fallen out of favour in the timeframe of the research project: 'they did learn from the experience of gene therapy, don't push it too much because of the backlash ... a lot of the scientists were unhappy with that ... nobody wants their work to be ... discredited or trashed' ('Lucy'); 'after billions of dollars and a decade of orchestrated hype from the biotech–medical industry, there is no gene therapy that has worked' (DAA 2005); It is often remarked in the context of genetics, that hype has a quasi-religious ring to it: 'Many writers make grand claims for science – that it is the new "religion" that it holds all the answers for the future and that scientists are the new "power elite"' (DAA 2005); 'Genetics offers redemption' ('James'); 'There's been a lot of messianic handwaving about gene therapy, but it'll be a while before they sort out the delivery problems' (Molecular biologist in personal email, 2004).

We have seen that the media also plays a role in hype such as in over-playing the 'breakthrough' card (chapters 1 and 2), and how the pharmaco industry and associated players in the 'bio-economy' have also hyped future outcomes. Chapter 4 discussed how the future promise of genetics is also one of 'bio-economic' promise; a golden economic future for individuals, companies and countries that invest in this bio-technology revolution. Subsequently economic competition, together with an articulated need for speedy responses in this area of 'rapid progress', underlies an imperative to strike while the iron is hot. UK and EU policy has been consistently shown to favour economic imperatives in relation to human genetics and bioscience generally. The promissory discourses of the bio-economy are a form of economic 'futures trading'; invest in this, and there will be economic and health rewards. Some sceptics consider that future 'winners' will be those who share in profits, and that cures and treatments in fact play second fiddle to economic criteria. Some argue that market forces are moulding the shape of the developments along specific lines, and that economic imperatives have led to the aggressive marketing of genetic/genomic futures (hype). Thus future genetic outcomes are based on economic imperatives; pharmacogenomics products for rich Western 'bio-consumers' is the subject of more research investment than third world disease.

In describing the operation of the bio-economy as a type of 'futures trading', one notes how stock market prices vary according to the perceived (bio) value of products, services and resources. The value of shares in 'big pharma' or any part of the bio-economy can go down as well as up, as the phrase goes. Like any other market investment, investment in bioscience is a gamble on future promissory benefits, predominantly financial rewards. Gambling metaphors pepper accounts of 'big pharma' strategies. There are financial risks as well as potential benefits, and financial risk appears to be dictating how players in the bio-economy are currently making moves.

[In] 2001, bio tech had a very high valuation based on the promise of the hype of genomics ... you're no longer able to raise fifty million dollars on the back of a genetics programme for Alzheimer's disease. Whereas that would have happened ... maybe five years ago. And it's well documented, companies have raised very large amounts of money on a promise of what a genetics programme will deliver.

('Ian')

Such financial risk catalyses arguments from health and social justice campaigners about genetics research as 'bad value' and a waste of public money in relation to population health provision (chapter 6).

Much genetic 'future promise' talk invokes notions of progress. Bioscientific research is framed in terms of progress almost by default. Here is the pro research charity 'Progress Educational Trust' (PET):

[PET] believes that ... the development of IVF has already led to the birth of thousands of babies across the world. Genetic testing, carried out before or during pregnancy, has offered parents the chance to have children free from a particular genetic disease. Assisted reproduction and genetics offer an alternative to those who are unable – because of infertility or because they have a genetic disease in their family – to consider normal methods of having children. However, Progress Educational Trust believes that the public should be involved in discussion about these sometimes contentious issues.

(PET ca. 2008)

Despite the call for 'balanced public debate' on these issues, PET goes on to foreground successes and benefits of this technology in very specific contexts. The very use of the word 'progress' in its title means that PET lays claim to certain values and ways of doing things as being progress by default. But what exactly does progress consist of? Progress is not something one can sensibly be 'against'. To call someone anti progress is a slight. But, like other similar words, such as 'freedom', it is a normative concept which can mean all things to all people. When something is enrolled as progress this implies certain values, certain norms, and thus what counts as progress is context-dependent, subjective; based on one's 'lifeworld' view. To qualify as progress a specific technology or application must be some kind of benefit. But benefits are contested territory too; what constitutes a benefit? And what about the accompanying burdens that benefits might bring? Potential difficulties arise over many promised genetic advances. This relates to the staking of claims over what counts as 'the public good'.

I believe that the vast majority of scientists do want to pursue progress to make the world a better place, my issue is that an equal number see science as the *only* way to gain betterment. I would argue this not to be the case.

(Email on chat list accessed by the author, 2005)

Those who are labelled as 'anti progress' are often slammed as Luddites. However they generally simply have different notions of what progress involves, and/or may be proceeding with differing degrees of caution. People voicing concerns do not necessarily wish to stop medical or genetic developments, but to warn or advise that concomitant changes – some more predictable than others – will come with those developments, and that these need to be accommodated, thought through, planned for, possibly prevented. Various campaign groups have responded vigorously to this highly charged use of words, and how it 'frames' them: 'That binary opposition comes up so much, you're for or against technology, you're for or against progress, it's used in practice to ridicule, to stifle debate' ('Lucy'). There are concerns that progress in one area might lead to backward steps in others: e.g. that progress in eliminating genetic disabilities might lead to greater stigma for those who do have disabilities versus hope that it will release greater resources for these people. This fits into a general fear that concentrating on specific types of 'genetic progress' will lead us to ignore social progress, for example issues of equity and access; or that social inequalities may in fact be exacerbated (chapter 6). Activists critical of the way human genetics futures are being constructed want to emphasise their own accounts of progress (which could of course include a role for genetics too) – social justice, equal access, eradicating poverty – as routes to health provision.

Utopias and dystopias: enhancement and transhumanism

All accounts of the future are based on present-day norms and values, whether implicitly or explicitly. These are a mix of individuals' personal perspectives, and the influence of values of particular systems, societies and their political and cultural practices, 'ways of doing things'. Using the example of transhumanism and enhancement, this final section shows how some commonly heard framings of utopias and dystopias invoke a specific future based on specific values and viewpoints.

A publication by the UK think tank Demos comprising an edited collection of chapters on enhancement provides a useful overview of different positions currently being articulated by civil society (Miller and Wilsdon 2006). Transhumanists[3] tend to provide a list of 'usual suspect' traits which could be 'enhanced'; performativity, longevity, intelligence, beauty. This in itself says something about the values they hold; enhancing compassion, for example, is not something one hears transhumanists making a case for. Such claims invoke the future, and are generally made on behalf of others, specifically future generations. At its most vivid, there are visions (or warnings) that enhancement that will be differentially distributed. Some have suggested the possibility that the human species may split in two, into the 'gene rich' and the 'gene poor' (Silver 1997). How people react to this idea says something about their values. A further value inherent in transhumanism futures talk is a highly favourable construction of science and technology as the key means by which society, the human race, will progress (Roco and Bainbridge 2003).

The key values debate inherent in such enhancement talk is what someone means by 'better' people; what counts as enhancement, and is this in any case a good thing? Life extension, for example, may cause social problems and widen existing inequalities; people living longer uses up resources. Enhancement discourse sails very close to notions of eugenics: specific characteristics are seen as having value; in some people's accounts, to enhance intelligence is progress; and to screen out disability, for example Down's syndrome, is also progress.

Trans- and post-human accounts of future enhancement tend to draw on very detailed, complex technical accounts of what might be possible and how it might be possible; smart drugs, bio and nano-engineered uploads for cognitive processes. The science is seen as so unlikely by some 'watchdogs' that they resist forecasting the implications of enhancement:

> I don't think anyone will be to be able to be enhanced ... the idea that you're going to have a separate 'gene rich' species I think is problematic if you start arguing against it, because I think you give credence for the scientific power.
>
> ('Jenny')

However other prime movers have grasped the nettle; they say that the science may be unlikely, but the signs point in specific directions, and so they are mobilising pre-emptively to forecast risks and threats. These prime movers are thus not focusing on whether the science is possible, or whether people have a 'right to choose' it, but rather on a political and economic analysis which examines the marketing of specific values, as this advert for a 2005 workshop co-hosted by the watchdog ETC group and the Dag Hammarskjold Foundation demonstrates:

> Genomics ... promises to ... 'enhance human performance'. In the current dominant trend of commodification of all aspects of life, everything and everybody can be 'improved' to increase consumption of corporate products or enhance military power. Drugs targeted for particular racial groups is one of the many problematic aspect of genomics research as are eugenic attempts to eliminate the disabled and diverse.[4]

This is a very politically situated account of enhancement as (bio) discrimination and commodification, and was repeatedly brought up by prime movers such as 'Mike': 'that idea of human enhancement and needing to technologically enhance ourselves, runs across genetics, genomics, nano-tech … it's very much a strategy by the pharmaceutical industry' ('Mike'). Similarly, Habermas (2003) refers to 'market-led eugenics'. This is not eugenics in the sense of state-led programmes, but rather a market-led, liber-alised eugenics which encourages specific 'choices' to enhance a particular trait (intelligence, beauty). Cosmetic surgery is a key indicator of where the tech-nology would go if it could; for example, R&D and media coverage has focused on the potential use of stem cells for breast 'enhancement', immedi-ately blurring the boundaries between medical and cosmetic use.[5]

Disability Rights campaign groups in particular also combine an alternative account of values with a political analysis of power stakes. The following quotation is from a press release by a group calling itself People Against Eugenics relating to a protest event about the use of reproductive technolo-gies, held at the Royal Society in 2004: 'Disabled people are human beings too – a "healthy" nation is one in which difference is included and celebrated – not a nation designed by the powerful' (PAE 2004). Thus enhancement discourse, ostensibly about the future, is very much about the values people hold in the here and now, and this is an important way of approaching the debate: 'the idea of enhancing ourselves would seem to be having completely the wrong anthropology … Because what really needs to evolve is the moral and spiritual aspect, and societal and relational, not whether you're intelligent' ('James').

'Science fiction' has long been a literary genre which has engaged with bio-scientific themes, using an imagined future to locate issues in an all-too-real-present. The future and the science are settings for some things the author wants to say, to bring to life, to reflect, about the human condition, and contemporary society. Several contemporary novelists are using future set-tings in their novels to discuss values issues raised by ideas of the trans- or post-human. One of the most well known is Margaret Atwood's 2003 novel *Oryx and Crake*. Three other novels which draw on bioscience themes are: Tim Pears' *Wake up* (2002), David Mitchell's *Cloud Atlas* (2004) and Kazuo Ishiguro's *Never Let Me Go* (2005). All three novels draw on human repro-ductive cloning as a viable reality.

In *Cloud Atlas* and *Never Let Me Go*, human clones are imagined by the authors as being created specifically for social functional purposes; clones in *Cloud Atlas* in a future some hundred years from now do the menial labour, are specifically bred to function in specific environments such as radioactive ones, or to be playthings of the super-rich. In *Never Let Me Go*, chillingly set in a contemporary present, clones are bred as spare parts for humans. *Wake Up*, conversely, also set in the present, tells the story of an infertile man, a maverick businessman, who has had himself cloned to provide himself and his wife (who successfully gives birth to this baby) with offspring. The clone in this book is thus envisaged as a valued child whereas the other two tell stories about clones created as functional objects. *Wake Up*, perhaps the most 'rea-listic' novel, also sets cloning in the ('real life') social environment where such an action is against the law. In contrast, in *Cloud Atlas* and *Never Let Me Go*, cloning is a socially sanctioned reality; clones in fact exist to serve society and are defined as sub-human.

All three novels address the issue of value, and human nature – what it means to be human. *Never Let Me Go* and *Cloud Atlas* both imply that clones should have value, be accorded 'human rights' denied them by the societies they were created to serve. Issues of citizenship are very important; the clones in *Never Let Me Go* and *Cloud Atlas* talk heartbreakingly of how it is their 'duty' to serve society. Embedded here is the idea that such discourses of citizenship can be bent to mean anything at all, depending on who is doing the defining. Both authors address, with a highly sinister twist, the power relations underpinning such descriptions of what 'duty' signifies. The unfairness and lack of social justice in creating beings which are treated in such a way is one level of meaning; at another, the philosophical idea of what being human *means* is also addressed, in very subtle nuances, felt as much as understood, by the reader. What all authors tackle, though, is the sense of individual identity, worth, value, and how status – even the status of 'human' – is something which is socially constructed, and individually felt.

Cloud Atlas and *Wake Up* both tackle 'consumer culture', identifying that we get the science we deserve; the science applications are developed to perform to society's desires. The 'the only place is out in front' brashness of the anti-hero in *Wake Up* is an identifiable type, one who would clone if he or she could, and who has the resources to make it happen. The vacuous, image-conscious, shallowly superficial society envisaged by the author of *Cloud Atlas*, whilst the most 'sci fi', is a depiction of contemporary consumer culture. The 'genomed generation' in *Cloud Atlas* is exhorted to consume, in fact consumption is another social 'duty'.

Conclusion

This chapter has provided some examples of different sorts of 'futures talk', showing how the future is invoked, in what contexts, and why this is significant. Constructions about where genetics is going or could go arise out of people's present worldview; their political analysis, their values and beliefs, in relation to the world they inhabit (and/or, frame themselves as inhabiting), in the present moment in time. The meanings people give to genetics in the here and now (not least, the credence they give to the viability of the vaunted science) influence the way in which they invoke the future. Further, specific invocations of the future catalyse public responses; people respond to perceived threats and opportunities. We have seen that values are normative, and hence accounts of progress and future benefits associated with specific applications and techniques are more contested than might at first appear. One person's risk is another's benefit; the enhanced post-human, for example. There are identifiable hierarchies of power and also of interest;

certain groups, political systems, and economic pressures, are framing the future along a specific axis; uneven power relations are framing specific futures. We have seen that the future promise of cures and treatments in particular has a tendency to drown out other concerns, such as risk. Such futures talk thus has profound health and social policy implications; the discourse itself is performing the future into being. It is imperative that there is a level playing field for different ideas of what the future should be like.

Conclusion

Locating human genetics debates

The book has drawn on (primarily UK-based) narratives; stories, arguments, interviews, and other evidence of social mobilisation as diverse as protest activity, website data, or the contents of a consultation document, showing that in multiple arenas civil society is debating and engaging with human genetics. We have seen how different publics interact and relate to each other through different types of network activity; transferring and contesting knowledge and information between each other, through a continual process of debates, conversations, involvement in consultations and a myriad of other interactions. The meanings of human genetics which people construct in these ways are being materialised into social realities, as different publics make use of resources such as the media, lobby for research budget spends, form multiple forms of social 'assemblages'. The book has provided some narratives of the social co-construction of specific sites of 'techno-science', aiming to identify and analyse some of the different interconnecting threads of social engagement, and different levels of influence.

The book has aimed to describe the social landscape of human genetics. Locating the debates within political, environmental and social landscapes – identifying 'geographies of technology' – informs an understanding of 'where people are coming from' when they frame the issues. The book has drawn on 'green' politics literature to locate debates on health, identity and citizenship in a broader political landscape (Plows and Boddington 2006) beyond that of individualised bioethics, for example in relation to concepts of 'informed consent' (chapter 7). This literature has also informed the description of the primary case study group as 'sustainability citizenship' prime movers (Barry 2005), because their key frames of reference tend to relate to issues of environmental social justice, and accompanying critical evaluations of existing power relations. All publics 'locate' human genetics in various ways and at different scales, such as the individual and the community, the global and the local. In relation to 'the local', for example, people identify and negotiate genetic risks and benefits relating to themselves and their families, for example to test or not to test (chapter 5). They may discuss the impact of their local environment on their health and situate claims being made for genetically focused health outcomes in these terms (chapter 6). Global spaces are also important sites when thinking about the social, political and economic spaces in which human genetics is manifesting, and/or co-producing. Global and local are linked in many ways, and are framed as such by many publics, perhaps especially in environmental social justice accounts of the impacts of the global on the local, and vice versa. The emergent term 'glocal' (Eschle and Stammers 2005) describes this synergistic flow. Examples given in this book include the global flows and supplies of bio-material; for example, chapter 2 provided a narrative on how stem cell lines from specific bodies and times and places (Romania, India) become globalised commodities. Support for, and criticisms of, the 'bio-economy', discussed in chapter 4, are a key theme which underpins the social reality of bio-material as a globalised resource with ' bio-value' (Waldby 2002).

Routledge's (2003) concept of convergence spaces discussed in chapter 1, aids in locating human genetics debates and understanding what is happening when individuals, groups, institutions and so on come together in specific times and places to interact in different ways; to develop shared meanings, or to contest different knowledge bases. Convergence spaces will be very different, depending on the people, networks and institutions who create them, the issues which catalyse them and the reasons for coming together in them. It is in and through convergence spaces that people form hybrid alliances or draw lines. For example, the Down's syndrome protest at the prenatal testing conference discussed in chapter 5 was a deliberate attempt to open up a social space to Down's syndrome activists, who had been denied an opportunity to speak formally. The European Social Forum (chapter 1, Appendix 3) was another particular type of convergence space deliberately set up to develop capacity within 'alter globalisation' and Left-leaning networks, through running workshops on different issues including human genetics and science and society. Conversely, the 'convergence spaces' of the UK science and technology committee are much more fixed, rigid, hierarchical and permanent, less open, than other forms of social spaces, in the ways in which they perform certain frames and certain functions. This highlights the importance of political space (Foucault 2003; Rabinow 1996) in terms of understanding how the materialising of specific certain forms and framings of human genetics emerges out of well established political institutions. Understanding institutional space explains why public consultations on human genetics have a specific shape; they operate within a specific political landscape which shapes the ensuing public response.

The book has drawn together Science and Technology Studies literature on public engagement with science, with Social Movement Theory literature, to situate theoretically an understanding of how and why people mobilise, and what this signifies. For example, where and why people 'draw lines' in relation to specific issues can catalyse mobilisation, and examples given have included the storage of DNA of innocent people (chapter 3), or the conditions under which human eggs are collected for stem cell research (chapter 2). This literature has also informed an understanding of how identities are constructed and maintained and has enabled a thorough evaluation of the concept of 'public engagement', differentiating between policy-led practice and grassroots 'social movement'. This also informed the methodology for the project on which this book has been based (chapter 1). It has also ensured that public engagement has been a well interrogated concept throughout the book; for example critically examining the phenomena of bio-consumers who can be seen as both markets for goods and services, and also as new forms of 'patients' (chapters 4 and 5).

The book has also produced an account of 'the science' based on the narratives provided by the people producing and engaging with the science and the accompanying debates. Overviews have been given of human embryonic stem cell research, biobanking, testing and screening and pharmacogenomics, as well as many other aspects of techno-science such as bioinfomatics. It has aimed to set out, in lay terms, what 'the science' is generally said to consist of, what its goals are, and to what extent these are contested territory. This narrative is thus the result of acquired knowledge from the research data sites; namely from the accessed discourses (interviews, web material, publications) of the policy makers, scientific institutions and civil society 'prime movers' such as patient groups and genetic watchdogs, whose voices have been heard throughout the book. This account has aimed to enable a more informed reading of the narratives and debates being conducted about 'the science'. In the process, this narrative has highlighted that many of these techno-scientific processes are contested territory where meanings and end goals shift. The introduction also raised the point that while the book's examples of human genetics research and (actual or potential) applications may 'date' (though many examples given in the book are still very much emergent in the public sphere), to be too concerned about this 'dating' is to miss the point. The book has taken some snapshots of a landscape which is socially significant at this moment in time. It is important to document some of these techno-scientific social geographies as they emerge, and are engaged with, by different publics.

Multiple publics: assemblages and identity politics

Multiple publics have been shown to be engaging with human genetics. The book does not claim to provide a definitive map, but rather to have taken some snapshots in a complex field, in the process identifying some interesting and important patterns and providing some analysis of what these signify. Social actors form multiple 'hybrid objects' associated with different aspects of human genetics; Irwin and Michael (2003) describe these social convergence patterns as 'assemblages', and these patterns also reflect Deleuze and Guattari's (1987) descriptions of 'rhizomic' network activity. The field as a whole is characterised by network fluidity, the constant creation and bio-degrading of assemblages, including ones catalysed by gear shifts in the 'bio-economy' (chapter 4). We have seen that where different publics converge, and where they draw lines in the sand, context arend issue specific; for example the 'strange bedfellows' Hands Off Our Ovaries! campaign which emerged over the use of women's eggs in stem cell research (chapter 2). A more formalised example are the many kinds of hybrid assemblages of scientists and policy makers, such as the UK stem cell network Human Embryonic Stem Cell Coordinators (chapter 2), who are co-constructing policy frameworks and setting the regulatory agenda, and the 'co-laboratories' (Glasner and Rothman 2004) of public–private partnerships.

There are also significant sticking points. Power relationships and ingrained 'ways of doing things' can mean closed doors, one-way information and network flows, and very narrow terms of reference for identifying relevant stakes and stakeholders. Some network relationships between spheres and actor groups are thus more fixed and hierarchical – 'tree-like' – (Deleuze and Guattari 1987) than others; such as formalised policy processes whereby certain high profile scientists are often to be found on regulatory 'expert stakeholder' panels, but other groups find it difficult to gain access at all. The regulatory sphere is a more formalised space which is not as open to re-framing the terms of engagement as civil society stakeholders would often like. Further, economic discourses of competitiveness and deterministic accounts of genetic 'progress', linked to promissory bio-futures, also direct social traffic in a one-way flow (chapter 8).

What all these types of social assemblages highlight clearly is that complex forms of new 'identity politics' are emerging (Epstein 2004, 2007) embedded in people's lives, bodies, communities, as genetic meanings are enrolled and constructed to provide explanations of self. These have been theorised as types of 'bio-socialities' (Rabinow 1996; Rose 2001), as 'bio-citizenship' (Rose and Novas 2004) and in terms of public engagement (Wynne 2006; Welsh *et al.* 2007). There are some already very well established publics mobilising over genetic identities and meanings. In particular, many patient groups have mobilised over genetic explanations of specific disease. Some of these have been catalysed into being specifically through genetic/genomic discoveries. Other patient groups have incorporated genetic narratives into their pre-existing repertoires, mobilising to support new forms of medical research. There is no doubt that many publics are mobilising directly as a result of human genetic technologies and this is how Rabinow's concept of 'bio-socialities' can be understood. However individual and collective identities are hugely contested territory; while identities are being constructed and understood through genetics by some, they are also seen as under threat from the meanings given to genetics by others, especially in relation to debates about what constitutes health, and health policy. Many identify a major risk of 'geneticisation' (chapter 6), which can be summarised as the reification of identity through the privileging of a specific construction of genetic meaning. Certain groups are in fact having to mobilise to protect challenges to their identity and community triggered by the construction of genetic meanings;

for example, Di Chiro (2008) shows how marginalised communities living in polluting environmental conditions are contesting research which potentially frames them as having 'genetic susceptibility' to pollution (chapter 6).

The theorist Melucci discussed the process through which social movements develop a 'collective identity' (1996). Individuals and even groups have been shown throughout the book to be constructing or contesting genetic meanings in relation to their identity. Defining publics in terms of their bio-identities has been shown to be sticky territory. Identity is an exceptionally complex and difficult topic in relation to human genetics; plural, fluid and contested identities, new forms of 'identity politics', rather than 'collective identities', characterise public engagement with human genetics (Plows 2008a). Chapter 1 and chapter 6 identified that concepts of bio-identities need strong interrogation; is the bio-frame the best means to understand complex 'identity politics'? In Plows and Boddington (2006) a critique was made of Rose and Novas's term 'bio-citizens', namely that the bio-label is often a reductive framing for identity claims and stakes, and one which has a tendency to ' frame out' – that is, not refer to – the social, political, and economic context of how such bio-identities are created in the first place. There are multiple identity claims and identity fragmentations, for example between and within patient and Disability Rights groups. Responses can vary from a straightforward identification with a genetic syndrome, to lobbying for treatments and cures. Rose and Novas's discussion of 'bio-citizens' specifically relates to patient groups who are mobilising in relation to human genetics, and are predominantly framing promissory discourses of genetics and framings of their identities in terms of genetic conditions. However, others are rejecting a geneticised framing of their identity; Disability Rights groups emphasise a social and political re-location of themselves as social actors.

Complex 'identity politics' debates and constructions thus need to be grounded in concepts of social justice and equity as much as genetically led discourses, when discussing questions of health, identity and accruing citizenship stakes; this is a policy issue, and this debate has been central to the book. Further, vested interest is affecting genetic identity construction. Many say that there is a market-led construction of bio-identities. There are identifiably bio-consumers who are shopping for bio-identity, within a marketplace where being 'genetically predisposed' to a certain trait may have only the most tenuous relevance, depending on the specific test. Chapter 4, for example, discusses the issue of 'syndrome invention', and chapter 5 details the commercial availability of genetic test kits.

Community is also an important concept in relation to identity and public engagement, especially when thinking about public engagement in terms of network relationships. The importance of community is reflected in the concept of community benefit-sharing, identified in bio-ethics discourse (chapter 3). Not only are there questions about what counts as a benefit, there are also questions around the definition of community. Where are the boundaries and borders? Who defines who is in or out? Concepts of genetic communities and disease communities many be of use (chapter 5); a genetic community may have very localised links, as specific genetic expression may be linked to certain geographical sites. A 'disease community' consisting of people with a specific genetic condition is also likely to be globally located.

Framing the debates

If the book is a little confusing, this is perhaps as it should be. Things *are* confusing, because they are complex. Ambivalence is an identifiable and important phenomenon in complex social sites, and the job of the social scientist is to find ways of exploring and explaining this 'mess', as Law (2006) points out; not to reify and simplify narrative lines down to 'one size fits all' neat boxes. Ambivalence is also likely to be characteristic of a still-emergent social field; even 'prime movers and early risers' are still in a process of working out what the stakes of the debate are (Welsh *et al.* 2007). Many people display ambivalence even when they hold very strong views on certain issues; often, they can observe that risks and benefits are tied together, identifying the 'burden of choice' in relation to prenatal testing, for example (chapters 5, 7). Even though we can arrive at better understandings of what stakes are relevant through being aware of the many discourses being articulated, these are not fixed and they will shift, morph and develop; this is the co-construction of meanings in action. The book has not set out to provide definitive stakes; it has provided some pointers, turned over some different stones in a very muddy social field.

The book has identified that there are plenty of situations in which the debates are being framed, by specific actors, in 'pro and anti' terms; such as 'for or against' embryonic stem cell research, or 'for or against' 'the right to choose'. However while acknowledging that these pro and anti debates do reflect 'real' positions, the book has also shown that in reality these are often overly polarised, and often very unhelpful ways of conducting debates on complex issues. It is this framing of the debate which is a main point of contention for many:

> the point is not to put the gene in the centre; the point is to look at what is it to talk about social justice, and therefore what roles does any of the genetics play in it, we determine the framework first and then we see if you fit ... rather than the framework, the questions being determined and you're just responding back because you cannot discuss therefore what is outside the framework.
>
> ('Lucy')

Horlick-Jones, Walls and Kitzinger (2007) discussed the ways in which literate publics 'read' the media by bringing their experiences to bear in their constructions and deconstructions; a process they term 'bricolage'. However while identifying that many publics are highly reflexive about the ways the debates are being framed, it is also the case that others – a key example perhaps being the burgeoning phenomenon of 'bio-consumers' shopping for an increasing range of genetic tests of questionable accuracy – may be less reflexive about the social realities they are co-constructing into being and the market forces and discourses which are catalysing their actions. It may also be the case, as identified in chapter 5, that patient groups and other citizens faced with making 'difficult choices', especially women in the context of reproduction and genetic testing, may not be as aware as they could be of the background social, political and economic forces at work, individualising the responsibility of their 'choice'. Women in the UK who are routinely prenatally screened for Down's syndrome unless they 'opt out' (chapter 5) are perhaps the thin end of a rapidly widening wedge.

Importantly, the book has also identified that often when people are ostensibly talking about human genetics, generally what is happening is that – catalysed by an issue such as genetic testing or stem cell research – people are framing this issue in terms of a range of other issues and values which are important to them and make sense in their own 'lifeworlds', which they see the specific catalyst issue as affecting. 'Adrian' reflects this when he says: 'if the framework which science is working in [is] a neo liberal version of a market economy where the rich get richer and the poor get poorer, you are going to get the one version of human genetics' ('Adrian'). These values themselves generally have subjective and contested meanings (for example, justice, choice), and certainly multiple methods of achieving these goals, which can predispose actors to be talking at cross-purposes past each other, often needlessly.

Trying to navigate some paths through this tangle of discourses, the book has aimed to identify recurring themes which stay consistent through many seemingly different issues and examples. The book has shown how many different debates about human genetics exist, and that they often run in parallel lines. This has hopefully made some of the important interconnections between these different trains of thought more explicit. Key frames such as hope for cures and treatments, and 'bigger picture' themes such as health and power, consistently emerge in the debates or are implicit within them, whether the context is stem cells or DNA databases. The ownership and use of bio-material and its privatisation have also been shown to be contested topics in a number of different contexts. The specifics of course do shift; issues of risk or benefit are different in different cases, but the concept of risk, for example, stays constant.

Promissory discourses in relation to human genetics are multiple and complex. The most common frame, and a consistent theme across different genetic sites, is hope for cures and better management of disease. Partially through the narrative of 'the science itself' accompanying chapters 2–5, the book has provided many examples of how human genetics R&D in many different ways is aiding in the understanding of different disease expression, and showing how different actors – scientists, policy makers and patient groups in particular – are saying that such work may provide cures and treatments in the future. Situated narratives of the many different types of people who need cures and treatments for diseases have thus been given, including stories of patient groups and others who are mobilising very effectively on the public stage to support R&D with regard to a number of genetically informed applications. For example, the book has provided first-hand accounts of the support for stem cell research and pharmacogenomics by patient groups with family members affected by serious diseases such as Cystic Fibrosis (chapter 2). 'Alice' and 'Ian' provide different narratives of the promise of their scientific research; for example, 'Alice' discusses her motivation to conduct open-source research (chapter 4).

The book has also identified that promissory accounts of benefits are not straightforward (chapter 8). For example, what are seen benefits for some could be seen as risks for others, such as the increase in prenatal tests available and the issue of the 'slippery slope' (chapter 5). Having genetic information is not necessarily a straightforward benefit though it is framed this way in certain contexts, for example by the genomic text kit provided by '23 and me' (chapter 5). Chapter 8 discussed the idea that 'futures talk' is very much about their values and social expectations in the here and now. What is really at stake for people? Issues of health, security, happiness are highly personal values; beauty is truly in the eye of the beholder. There are politically orientated frames of promissory economic futures too; the promise is that human genetics will deliver economic advantage for nation states; for example, 'UK plc'. Hope can be seen to become hype especially in relation to economic performativity and the performance of the 'future science', for example in the discourses of and about 'big pharma' (chapter 4). Importantly, different developments in genetics and bioscience, whether gene therapy, stem cells, pharmaco and so on, are accompanied by highly promissory discourses from a number of sources, but have not delivered much in the way of reliable end products beyond the continuing expansion of the test-as-product (chapter 5, chapter 6). 'Future promise' (Brown and Michael 2003) narratives of cures and progress need to be examined, located, more critically.

'Sustainability citizenship' actors such as 'Lucy' and 'Mike' tilt the frame, taking the eye away from the future promise as viewed down the genetics lens, and locating debates about health in the broader context of social and environmental justice. In doing so, they are re-framing the question implicit in many human genetics debates – what is health and how can we be healthy? Rather than talk about prolonged life expectancy in terms of genetic enhancement for the few, for example, they will discuss how life expectancy can be enhanced for the many through the provision of safe, clean environments. Many examples are given in the book of how campaign groups and networks are trying to shift the terms of the debates on human genetics and shed a different light on what is at stake. Identity, equality, individualised responsibility and the role of market forces have also been important points of entry into the debates for these groups. By providing examples of their narratives and actions, the book has aimed to broaden the perspective of the genetics lens, and thus to introduce dimensions which are often 'framed out' of these debates.

> Minatec will be ... Europe's most important research, teaching and implementation center on nanotechnologies. ... social and urban harms ... are bound to get worse: creation of an Isère Silicon Valley, fast increase of rents and traffic jams, soaring prices, mass arrivals of executives drawing away the poors to the suburbs.
> (Activists in Grenoble France occupy construction site for Minatec Nanotech centre 2004-12-13.)[1]

The quotation above frames the issues at stake in the 'lifeworlds' of some specific activists, in relation to the Minatec nanotech R&D centre in Grenoble. They literally locate the debate in its socio-geographical context.

Watchdogs such as GeneWatch and ETC group are amongst those critical of the fact that powerful actors such as the bio-tech industry deliberately frame the potential future of human genetics in specific ways, in terms of things which have value to people, such as their future health, often in order to market their specific product, but dis-located from political, economic, social and environmental contexts such as the fact that poverty predisposes to ill health. They also argue that 'market-led science' is constructing markets of people framed as 'predisposed' to disease, rather than actively seeking to develop holistic health policies (chapter 4 and 6).

Whose human genetics? Public engagement, citizenship and agenda setting

A key critique consistently raised by many prime movers has been that the policy debates in particular are set by powerful elites, in very taken-for-granted ways of doing things which narrow down, reify and polarise important issues. Examples include what is left out of policy consultations, or how what is put into them frames the debate a certain way, emphasising the importance of which words are used and how some words come to be used ('choice', for example, in relation to egg sourcing; chapter 7). These different actors and institutions and 'ways of doing things' (such as UK public engagement consultation processes) 'frame' the debating process and thus co-construct not only the sorts of debates about human genetics which are had, but also the shape of the genetics itself and the way it impacts on the social sphere, the social landscape. Further, research agendas with specifically envisioned applications at UK, EU and international levels can be heavily influenced by powerful lobby groups which prioritise certain sorts of research into certain arenas (Birch 2006).

This process further performs social reality and social 'truth' about the meanings and shape of human genetics into being. It is in these processes that some discourses and actions become solidly performed and often reified, whereas others fade away, only heard in very different social spheres and spaces which are usually not seen as relevant to the 'main debate' – the dominant set of knowledge claims and meanings – or if they are, often mis-understood, misrepresented or sidelined. During the research for this book, an NGO prime mover spoke of her experiences of being in policy/industry meetings about genetics, wanting to talk about social policy and health, and being told that she was effectively 'in the wrong meeting'. This reification and exclusion process happens even when it is well understood by a range of powerful actors. Power relations thus affect what stakeholders get to sit at the policy table. Some civil society and academic success can be claimed through the fact that awareness of this has filtered through to policy level, where moves have been made to include a broader range of stakeholders 'upstream' in the debates (Wilsden and Willis 2004; Wynne 2006). A loudly heard counter-argument is that 'upstream' is still very much 'downstream' in terms of agenda-setting:

> Demos has ... produced a report, See Through Science, that calls on industry, government and scientists to involve concerned groups in shap-ing research into problematic subjects such as nanotech at a much earlier stage than commercialisation. The problem with this argument is that for a development to be seen as 'concerning' ... usually happens well after industry and government have set their targets.
>
> (Corporate Watch 2005)

With this in mind, carving out some political space for themselves outside of the policy sphere, other social actors eschew the political arena altogether and opt for the 'upstream public engagement' approach of protest, such as the Grenoble anti Minatec activists already cited:

> potential consequences and benefits drawn by research can't be nor debated nor controlled by the populations ... Shutting this site ... is attempting to stop a project that we refuse. It's an opportunity to launch once again the idea of a necessary social change, here and elsewhere. To stop and think. It seems to us essential to interrupt development's headlong rush.

Mobilisation outside of the public sphere, including such 'confrontational' direct action, flags up the fact that in many cases 'stakeholders' are not being invited to form policy, or where relevant stakeholders have been identified and enrolled, their presence and influence is minimal, not to say token. And this is because power relations and their effects on knowledge and expertise claims making and staking do not simply determine who gets to be a stakeholder. Power relations determine *who sets the stakes in the first place*; identifying what is seen as central to the debate. Thus some 'stakeholders' are bound to have more legitimacy in this practice, while other groups do not even get defined as stakeholders at all.

To reiterate, stating that pro genetics research patient groups are favoured by policy and industry is not a conspiracy theory, it is a simple statement of fact. Nor is this statement of fact necessarily to criticise the values and goals of these actors. It is however important to consider which futures are being framed out or never conceived of – at least by those in power – in these processes. It is here where debates about health policy and strategies, especially in relation to discourses of sustainable development, social and environmental justice and equity, are at their most relevant. Grassroots community groups and NGOs are experts in these arenas (chapter 6) and their voices need to be heard more loudly in debates about health strategies. They argue that a wealth of relevant knowledge on community health policy and environmental justice is often left out of the frame when the promises of specific forms of bioscience are being vaunted. They also say that budget spends of nations are being affected, noting that there are risks attached when health policy is set in terms of overly promissory genetic/genomic discourses, for example the World Health Organisation (WHO 2005) also critiques genetic hype in the context of disease prevention (chapter 8).

The attempts to enrol more stakeholders 'upstream' are linked to debates about citizenship; that citizens should have the option of inputting into policies which will affect them. Specific discourse on human genetics, including from policy makers, has been shown to make strong claims on citizenship and altruism; to enrol concepts of rights, duties and choices; for example, in relation to the donation of bio-material (chapters 2, 3 and 6). The book has shown that these calls to public altruism have been challenged on several counts, including assessment of differentially experienced risks and questioning of who benefits and how. Many, particularly 'sustainability citizenship' prime movers, have also been concerned about the trend towards individualised responsibility and even blame in relation to ones health, as Di Chiro's assessment (2008) of the implications of susceptibility genes for environmental justice, discussed in chapter 6, demonstrates. There are those who are (blamed and) framed, and there are those doing the framing. The framed may and do resist, of course, and their stories have been told in this book, for example those at risk of suffering genetic discrimination or those Disability Rights activists who feel their value as human beings is at stake through what they see as eugenics policies. These and other struggles over identity and citizenship are set against a backdrop of powerful elites and knowledge claims. Many point out that technology both (re) produces, and is itself a product of, existing social patterns, inequalities and power structures, and it is this issue of the 'politics of technology' which they identify as needing discussion. They are raising questions about the relationship between science and society: in what type of society do we want to live, and by what norms and values should it be driven?

> what we need to get to is … the politics of new technologies … that people can engage with, so that we're not dealing with nuclear power and then dealing with genetic engineering and then dealing with … those … separate local little areas … [but] to have a real live politics of how new technologies impact on society, how society has some control over that.
>
> ('Mike')

However publics simply cannot help but respond to specific issues raised by 'the next thing', because these new developments clearly have an impact on their 'lifeworlds'. Chapter 1 and chapter 6 in particular noted that theories of 'bio-socialities' (Rabinow 1999) and 'biocitizenship' (Rose and Novas 2004) must take account of the power relations which are constructing bio-framings of identity and citizenship stakes including responsibilities, duties (Plows and Boddington 2006) and individual 'choices' (chapters 5 and 7). The individualising of responsibility for health needs careful and critical interrogation; what will it mean to be a citizen in the light of geneticised accounts of health and identity and competing accounts and interests.

Conclusion: converging technologies, converging discourses

Some rapid developments have occurred in the biosciences in the timeframe 2003–7 covered by this book, such as the 'genomic turn' as much discourse shifted from genetics to genomics. Converging Technologies, sometimes referred to in terms of the disciplines they emerge from as 'Nano Bio Info Cogno'[2] are being framed as the 'next big thing' (Roco and Bainbridge 2003). Two core processes/end results in this next wave of techno-science are nano-biotechnology (nanobio) and synthetic biology (synbio). Both, in different ways, enrol a combination of biological and non-biological material, and biological material which has been 'artificially' created: 'Nanobiotechnology involves the integration of biological materials with synthetic materials to build new molecular structures or products' (ETC 2004). 'Researchers in an emerging field called synthetic biology envision microbes customized with artificial genes … a species of built-to-order bacteria using only man-made DNA' (Bloomberg 2008). Converging Technologies are new, but they have converging discourses (Plows and Reinsborough 2008); this is old wine in new bottles. Of course, specifically new bioscience developments and applications provide new landscapes to navigate. The risk of nanobio or synbio organisms loose in the environment poses new types of theoretical risks and uncertainties to the environmental risks and uncertainties posed by GM crops (ETC 2003). But the underlying issues still stay incredibly constant. Risk and power relations in this case are concepts which do not differ if the subject is GM crops, nanobio or nuclear power. There is very little which is new in the utopian/promissory or dystopian/risk discourses emerging in relation to Converging Technologies. There will be new actor groups emerging specifically in relation to these technologies but also there are highly significant social continuations, for example the patient groups and environmental/technology watchdogs already predisposed to mobilise because of their prior interest in these areas of science and the issues they raise.

Bucchi (2004) identified that 'cross talk' between different social groups such as 'scientists' and 'the public' is happening; the book has provided further examples of how discourses travel around social networks through the hybrid 'assemblages' which form either institutionally or more 'organically' in civil society. 'Cross talk' will occur on its own, and it can also be encouraged as part of governance processes. Currently the wealth of knowledge, the capacity, of different publics is not adequately reflected in the public debates and consultation processes. More needs to be heard about their experiences, their different types of expertise, and the ways in which they are framing genetics in terms of their own 'lifeworld' values and knowledge claims.

Policy-led accounts of public engagement need to develop understandings of how publics also create their own spaces for debate, and their own terms of those debates. This is not simply a methodological issue of getting more plural, more first-hand accounts of why publics are engaging, though this is certainly very important. It is a more politically situated account of what constitutes 'legitimate' public engagement. Currently, despite 'best practice' discourses of better public engagement, there is very little evidence that any of it translates into policy practice unless it fits with the agendas of elites. Further, power relations still clearly enable these elites to set agendas much more 'upstream' than other publics. January 2008 saw a set of emergent yet familiar promissory discourses on synbio performed by the influential scientist Craig Venter framing the debate along familiar tracklines of techno-fix 'future promise'; synbio is framed as a solution for, amongst other things, climate change.[3]

This book has aimed to provide a resource to understand how publics are debating and engaging with human genetics. It has identified, untangled and contextualised a number of different narrative threads. This has involved turning down the volume on some sets of discourses and turning up others, which are only faintly heard from the margins. There is no doubt that much of the social 'heat' is coming from patient groups wanting cures and treatments, a burgeoning strata of other bio-consumers (performing themselves into potential patients), scientists doing the science, industry, and policy. These voices can however frame the debates in certain ways which often unnecessarily polarise public debate, and hence the book has aimed to 'tilt the frame' to flag up the existence of other publics who often struggle to be heard. It is to be hoped that the book is a useful resource in the conducting of a holistic and constructive debate. It is also important to try to explore what ambivalence may actually signify in the domains of public engagement with genetics or bioscience more generally, and to recognise that taking a position in specific contexts doesn't necessarily mean that one is set against the position taken by another. While we are perhaps inevitably drawn to view 'through a glass, darkly' down the genetics lens, we can also appreciate the kaleidoscope of colourful, hybrid fragments which constitutes public engagement with human genetics.

Appendix 1: List of anonymised interviewees

Interviewees

All interviewed 2003–6 and UK-based

'Alice' – scientist specialising in bioinfomatics
'Lucy' – sustainable development watchdog spokesperson
'Jenny' – genetics watchdog spokesperson
'Susan' – patient group spokesperson
'Angela' – civil servant with genetics brief
'Jane' – patient group spokesperson
'Sally' – Disability Rights activist
'Mike'– technology watchdog spokesperson
'Ian' – science entrepreneur
'Dave' – 'green' anti capitalist activist
'James' – science and technology watchdog spokesperson
'Adrian' – 'green' campaigning journalist
'Peter' – patient charity spokesperson
'Dan' – 'green' anti capitalist activist

Appendix 2: List of acronyms and their website references

Acronyms

ACMG *American College of Medical Genetics* www.acmg.net

ACPO *Association of Chief Police Officers* www.acpo.police.uk

AMRC *Association of Medical Research Charities* www.amrc.org.uk

ARC *Antenatal Results and Choices* www.arc-uk.org

ARCH *Action on Rights for Children* www.arch-ed.org

ASHG *American Society of Human Genetics* www.ashg.org

BBSRC *Biotechnology and Biological Sciences Research Council* www.bbsrc.ac.uk

BERR *Department for Business, Enterprise & Regulatory Reform* www.berr.gov.uk

BICA *British Infertility Counselling Association* www.bica.net

BIS *(Department for) Business, Innovation and Skills* www.bis.gov.uk

CA *Consumers Association* www.Which.co.uk

CATs *Communities Against Toxics* www.communities-against-toxics.org.uk

CEC *Commission of the European Communities* http://ec.europa.eu

Cesagen *Centre for Economic and Social Aspects of Genomics* www.genomicsnetwork.ac.uk/cesagen/

CGS *Center for Genetics and Society* www.geneticsandsociety.org

CGS *Clinical Genetics Society* www.clingensoc.org

CMGS *Clinical Molecular Genetics Society* www.cmgs.org

CORE *Comment on Reproductive Ethics* www.corethics.org

CornerHouse *CornerHouse* www.thecornerhouse.org.uk

Corporate Watch *Corporate Watch* www.corporatewatch.org.uk

DAA *Disability Awareness in Action* www.daa.org.uk

DBIS *Department for Business, Innovation and Skills* www.bis.gov.uk

Defra *Department for Environment, Food and Rural Affairs* www.defra.gov.uk

DoH *Department of Health* www.dh.gov.uk

DRINC *Diet and Health Research Industry Club* http://www.bbsrc.ac.uk/business/collaborative_research/industry_clubs/drinc/index.html

DTI *Department of Trade and Industry* www.bis.gov.uk

EBI *European Bioinformatics Institute* www.ebi.ac.uk

EC *European Commission – see CEC*

EcoNexus *EcoNexus* www.econexus.info
EGC *the UK Biobank Ethics and Governance Council* www.egcukbiobank.
org.uk
EGE *European Group on Ethics* www.ec.europa.eu/european_group_ethics
EGP *Environmental Genome Project* www.niehs.nih.gov/research/supported/
programs/egp
EMBL *European Molecular Biology Laboratory* www.embl.org
EMEA *European Medicines Agency* www.emea.europa.eu
ESF *European Social Forum* www.fse-esf.org
ESRCGN *ESRC Genomics Network* www.genomicsnetwork.ac.uk
ESSF *European Science Social Forum Network* (no longer live)
ETC *Action Group on Erosion, Technology and Concentration* www.etcgroup.org
Ethox *Ethox Centre for medical ethics* www.ethox.org.uk
EU *European Union* see CEC
FINRRAGE *Feminist International Network of Resistance to Reproductive
and Genetic Engineering* www.finrrage.org
GAIC *Genetics and Insurance Committee* www.dh.gov.uk/ab/GAIC/index.htm
GeneWatch *GeneWatch* www.genewatch.org
GGD *Governing Genetic Databases* www.ethox.org.uk
GIG *Genetic Interest Group* www.gig.org.uk
GM Watch *GM Watch* www.gmwatch.eu
GTAC *Gene Therapy Advisory Committee* www.dh.gov.uk/ab/GTAC/index.htm
HESCCO *Human Embryonic Stem Cell Coordinators* www.ncbi.nlm.nih.gov/
pubmed/18154466
HFEA *Human Fertilisation and Embryology Authority* www.hfea.gov.uk
HGA *Human Genetics Alert* www.hgalert.org
HGC *Human Genetics Commission* www.hgc.gov.uk
HGP *Human Genome Project* www.ornl.gov/sci/techresources/Human_Genome
Home Office *Home Office* www.homeoffice.gov.uk
HOOO *Hands Off Our Ovaries* www.handsoffourovaries.com
HUGO *Human Genome Organisation* www.hugo-international.org
HUPO *Human Proteome Organisation* www.hupo.org
IoI *Institute of Ideas* www.instituteofideas.com
IPCB *Indigenous Peoples Council on Biocolonialism* www.ipcb.org
IPO *Intellectual Property Office* www.ipo.gov.uk
ISB *Institute for Systems Biology* www.systemsbiology.org
ISIS *Institute of Science in Society* www.i-sis.org.uk
ISSCR *International Society for Stem Cell Research* www.isscr.org
Liberty *Liberty* www.liberty-human-rights.org.uk
MHRA *Medicines and Healthcare Products Regulatory Agency* www.mhra.
gov.uk
MRC *Medical Research Council* www.mrc.ac.uk
MSF *Médecins Sans Frontières* www.msf.org.uk
NCB *Nuffield Council on Bioethics* www.nuffieldbioethics.org
NDNAD *UK police National DNA database* www.npia.police.uk/en/8934.htm

NESCI *North East England Stem Cell Institute* www.nesci.ac.uk

NICE *National Institute for Clinical Excellence* www.nice.org.uk

NIH *National Institute of Health*

NSC *National Screening Committee* www.screening.nhs.uk

NuGO *The European Nutrigenomics Organisation* www.nugo.org

OECD *Organisation for Economic Cooperation and Development* www.oecd.org

Patent Office (now the *Intellectual Property Office*) www.ipo.gov.uk

PET *Progress Educational Trust* www.progress.org.uk

PGD *Preimplantation genetic diagnosis*

PHG *Foundation Foundation for Genomics and Population Health* www.phgfoundation.org

PHM *People's Health Movement* www.phmovement.org

PICTF *Pharmaceutical Industry Competitiveness Task Force* www.advisorybodies.doh.gov.uk/pictf/

PND *Prenatal diagnosis*

PVMA *Patients' Voice for Medical Advance* www.patientsvoice.org.uk (apparently dormant, was SIMR)

PXE *PseudoXanthoma Elasticum patient group* www.pxe.org

ReproKult *ReproKult Frauen Forum Fortpflanzungsmedizin* www.reprokult.de

Royal Society *Royal Society* www.royalsociety.org

SACGT *Secretary's Advisory Committee on Genetic Testing* www.oba.od.nih.gov/SACGHS/sacgt_info.html

Sanger *Sanger Institute* www.sanger.ac.uk

SAS *Sense About Science* www.senseaboutscience.org.uk

sc4sm *Stem Cells for Safer Medicines* www.sc4sm.org

SIMR *Seriously Ill for Medical Research* see PVMA

TAC *Treatment Action Campaign* www.tac.org.za

TRIPS *Trade Related Intellectual Property Rights* www.wto.org/english/tratop_E/TRIPS_e/trips_e.htm

UK Biobank *UK Biobank* www.ukbiobank.ac.uk

UKGTN *UK Genetic Testing Network* www.ukgtn.nhs.uk

UKSCB *United Kingdom Stem Cell Bank*

UKSCF *UK Stem Cell Foundation* www.ukscf.org

UKSCI *UK Stem Cell Initiative* www.advisorybodies.doh.gov.uk/uksci/

UnCaged *UnCaged* www.uncaged.co.uk

UNESCO *United Nations Educational, Scientific and Cultural Organization* www.unesco.org

Wellcome Trust Biobank *see UK Biobank* www.ukbiobank.ac.uk

WHO *World Health Organization* www.who.int

WIPO *World Intellectual Property Organization* www.wto.org

WSF *World Social Forum* www.forumsocialmundial.org.br/index.php?cd_language=2

WTCHG *Wellcome Trust Centre for Human Genetics* http://www.well.ox.ac.uk/

WTO *World Trade Organisation* www.wto.org

Appendix 3: European Social Forum workshops

Human Genetics and Science and Society Workshops at the 2004 European Social Forum, London[1]

Human genetics/omics workshops:

1 *Developments in Human Genetics*

Organisation: GeneWatch UK, Human Genetics Alert, Institut Mensch Ethik und Wissenschaft, Gen Ethisches Network

2 *Bar coding people – Individualised health care or money making scam?*

Organisation: GeneWatch UK

3 *Human cloning and genetic engineering: what's at stake?*

Organisation: Human Genetics Alert

4 *Prenatal screening: eugenics or women's rights?*

Organisation: Human Genetics Alert

Related workshops-

Resisting corporate monopolies and new enclosures

Organisation: ETC group (Action Group on Erosion, Technology and Concentration), Green Party of Europe, Protimos

This was one of several workshops specifically on nanotechnology and Converging Technologies

Science and society workshops:

1 *What Research Policies Are Appropriate in Another Europe?*

2 *'Science and Citizenship'.*

3 *A European Science Social Forum*

[1] www.fse-esf.org/ (accessed 8 October 2009).

Notes

Introduction

1 Defined here as a certain set of technologies, applications and techniques – both actual and projected.
2 Every explanation of 'the science' is accompanied by a number of references to key scientific websites and studies, and readers are encouraged to check accounts given here through cross referencing.
3 'Early humans may have had help in mastering tools and walking upright from a chunk of DNA that scientists previously wrote off as junk' (*Guardian* 2008a) See also *New Scientist* (2008a).
4 Evans and Plows (2007) discuss how activists can become 'organic experts'.

1 Methodology and publics overview

1 A social movement as a specific form of collective behaviour has been defined by a number of social movement theorists as consisting of sustained collective protest activity over time, and the development of a movement 'collective identity' (Melucci 1996). It is possible that social movements are becoming more fragmented, fluid and complex; and that existing definitions of what a social movement *is* need updating to respond to changing social mobilisation patterns. Very little, if any, public engagement with human genetics can be defined as a social movement within the established definition of the term, even when specific groups such as patient groups or Disability Rights groups undertake protest activity. These are, however, socially significant important forms of mobilisation being taken by different publics. Here, the use of social movement theory represents a means of using an important set of sociological tools to describe and to understand public engagement with human genetics. For more discussion on this subject, see Plows (2008a).
2 Seattle 1999 was a decade ago and the controversy over G20 protests in London 2009 highlight that these protests are still an important repertoire of action.
3 YESS – Yearly European Science Society http://ec.europa.eu/research/conferences/2005/forum2005/showcase_yess_en.htm (accessed 18 June 2009).
4 'Café Scientifique is a place where, for the price of a cup of coffee or a glass of wine, anyone can come to explore the latest ideas in science and technology. Meetings take place in cafés, bars, restaurants and even theatres, but always outside a traditional academic context. Café Scientifique is a forum for debating science issues, not a shop window for science. We are committed to promoting public engagement with science and to making science accountable.' http://www.cafescientifique.org/ (accessed 16 June 2009).
5 Imperial College London Science Communication Group http://www3.imperial.ac.uk/humanities/sciencecommunicationgroup (accessed 15 February 2009).

6 Science Museum's Dana Centre http://www.danacentre.org.uk/ (accessed 15 February 2009).

7 Emerging Politics of New Genetic Technologies project http://www.lancs.ac.uk/fss/cesagen/politics/index.htm (accessed 15 February 2009).

8 Data examples were still being collated in 2007 and so there is no exact cut-off point between 2006 and 2007.

9 (Green Action 2004) Briefing for the European Peoples Global Action 2004 conference, held in Slovenia.

10 The 'anti globalisation movement' is a misnomer. Activists were not 'against globalisation' per se; they were in fact extremely globalised, for example, in their early use of the internet to develop international network links. Rather, these actors critiqued the specific type of globalisation linked to Neoliberal capitalist forms of economic competitiveness.

11 'The Rayner lab collaborates with other Sanger teams to use experimental genetic and proteomic approaches as well as novel protein–protein interaction tools to better understand the protein networks that drive the recognition, attachment and entry phases of (malarial) erythrocyte invasion.'
http://www.sanger.ac.uk/Teams/Team115/ (accessed 15 February 2009).

12 Commons www.parliament.uk/parliamentary_committees/ius.cfm (accessed 15 February 2009). Lords www.parliament.uk/parliamentary_committees/lords_s_t_select. cfm (accessed 15 February 2009).

13 the word ... breakthrough ... [is] over used ... but the stem cell transplant in Spain could be a significant step ... ' BBC Radio 4's 6 o'clock news, 19 November 2008.

2 Stem cells and cloning

1 In the USA the ban wasn't on the research, but on federal funding of it, prior to the Obama administration.

2 The extent to which this would actually be a complete genetic 'match' would vary, depending on the specifics of the technique. If the cell from a patient was used together with a donor egg, this would be a partial genetic match for the patient. If both the egg and the cell were derived from the (of necessity female) patient who was then also the recipient of the resulting treatment, this would constitute a complete genetic match.

3 http://www.genomicsnetwork.ac.uk/cesagen/events/pastevents/conferences/title,2929,en. html (accessed 15 July 2009).

4 see also the Joint committee on the Human Tissue and Embryos Bill which includes a chronology of relevant legislation, review and reports.

5 Cloning is a highly complex procedure. In cloning research for overcoming immune rejection, the nucleus is replaced specifically by a cell from a sick person, and more importantly, a differentiated cell, e.g. a skin cell. Until the 'breakthrough' of the cloned sheep Dolly, a differentiated cell was not believed to be able to differentiate back. Also replacing an egg with the nucleus of another cell doesn't itself create the cloned embryo. Further processes are needed before the constructed egg starts dividing as an embryo. This has been the point of challenges around the fact that the legal definition of an embryo is an egg and sperm, whereas a cloned embryo doesn't have any sperm.

6 During the 2007 UK Genomics and Society (EGN) conference, a 'Sense about Science' spokeswoman called regulatory frameworks 'unethical' because they slowed down research which might produce cures.

7 'During its first mandate the EGE (1998–2000) provided Opinions on subjects as diverse as human tissue banking, human embryo research, and human stem cell research ... During the second mandate period (2001–4), the Group widened the

scope of its ethical analyses producing Opinions on: patenting inventions involving human stem cells' (EGE 2005).

8 Stephen Minger of Kings College London was courting media attention in relation to hybrid embryos in 2006 on the back of the HFEA egg donor issue, claiming in radio interviews that his hybrid embryos were more 'ethical' and also more scientifically viable as a source of hESC than those derived from human eggs (Plows 2007b, 2008b).

9 Importantly, no payment is available for women 'altruistically donating', though they will get 'basic expenses' of £250.

10 A new sub-set of stakeholder 'patients' in relation to hES are the women undergoing IVF who may use 'egg-sharing' arrangements (Parry 2006) or women who may ' altruistically donate' eggs.

3 Biobanks and databases

1 Ensure 'your family are in a position to benefit from advances in regenerative medicine' (VHB 2008).

2 Annual Report (deCODE 2007). DeCode genetics filed for bankruptcy in November 2009 (*New York Times,* 17 November 2009).

3 'Did you ever wonder about your most ancient ancestors? The Genographic Project will introduce you to them' (Genographic Project 2008).

4 Annual Report (Celera 2008).

5 NIH (1990).

6 Sulston and Ferry (2002) produced a good lay guide to this epic project.

7 'GeneWatch UK believes that genetic horoscopes are a dangerous myth' (Gene-Watch 2009a).

8 Robert Terry is a Senior Policy Advisor at the Wellcome Trust, and here was speaking at the Genes and Society conference in April 2003.

9 The issue of 'right to access' genetic 'information' warrants critical examination. In the USA a lobby group have launched a campaign for your right to this (Health-DataRights 2009). An important question is whether access to information is meaningful in the absence of 'quality control' of that information.

10 'Intellectual property, income generation and royalties. Intellectual property and access policies are being developed to help ensure that the UK Biobank resource is accessible to all bona fide research users, but is not exploited improperly or used in any way that inappropriately constrains use by others. Terms of access will be embodied in legal agreements that reflect UK Biobank's objectives' (UK Biobank 2007).

11 'In medical research involving competent human subjects, each potential subject must be adequately informed of the aims, methods, sources of funding, any possible conflicts of interest, institutional affiliations of the researcher' (WMA 2008).

12 There are differences in (current, proposed) terms and conditions of DNA sample collation, storage and use between England/Wales, Scotland and Northern Ireland – see GeneWatch briefing for MPs (2007).

13 Annual Report, NPIA (2007).

14 DNA Expansion Programme, Home Office (2006).

15 0.5 per cent in the USA BBC (2006b).

16 '... A further 27,000 persons on the NDNAD who have not been charged or cautioned for any offence were under 18 years of age at the time they were arrested and had a DNA sample taken but had reached 18 by 1st December 2005 Hansard (2006b).

17 (GeneWatch *et al.* 2007).

18 'We also draw a clear distinction between the retention of the DNA profile (the "DNA fingerprint") on a computer and the original sample (the "CJ sample") in a freezer. The latter may potentially be retested and used in ways not considered

when it was originally taken. We welcome the Government's willingness to consider an independent oversight body for CJ samples' HGC (2002).

19 It is possible – though not easy or very transparent – to get oneself removed from the NDNAD without recourse to the courts (Register 2008) and in 2009 Gene-Watch organised a website, www.reclaimyourdna.org to make the process easier.

20 Author's notes, HGC plenary meeting September 2003.

21 The original press release that triggered this story came from the National Black Police Association (NBPA 2006).

22 See also *New Scientist* (2005b).

4 'PharmacoG' as product and process

1 For a 'user-friendly' overview of DNA and the role of proteins see, for example, Custer 2004.

2 Particularly 'Matrix Assisted Laser Desorption Ionisation' (MALDI); see Ashcroft 2009, ch. 6.

3 Interestingly, like 'pharmacoG', bioinfomatics is a loose term even amongst the scientific community and there is no standard definition. For example, http://www. biology.gatech.edu/graduate-programs/bioinformatics/new/whatis.php (accessed 17 April 2009).

4 See http://www.ornl.gov/sci/techresources/Human_Genome/faq/snps.shtml (accessed 6 Jun 2009) for an overview.

5 The 'mapping' metaphor is particularly questionable given the gaps in understanding relating to what sequenced bio-information actually signifies.

6 'Animals genetically modified and cloned for drug production (so-called "pharming")' (GeneWatch 2002a).

7 'Nutrigenomics is the science that examines the response of individuals to food compounds using post-genomic and related technologies (e.g. genomics, transcriptomics, proteomics, metabol/nomic etc.)' www.nugo.org/everyone/24023 (accessed 29 May 2009).

8 Nutriceuticals – plant-based production of pharmaceutical proteins http://hort.uark.edu/research-programs/nutriceuticals.html (accessed 6 June 2009).

9 'Nano products on the market: Promoting untested nano-technology Food and cosmetic companies are now collaborating to develop 'cosmetic nutritional supplements.' L'Oréal and Nestlé recently formed Laboratoires Innéov, a 50/50 joint venture. Innéov's first product, called 'Innéov Firmness,' contains lycopene. The supplement is taken orally and is marketed to women over 40 who are concerned about lost skin elasticity … the food and cosmetic alliances illustrate the tendency to blur boundaries between food, medicine and cosmetics, a trend that nanotech will likely accelerate' (Corporate Watch 2009).

10 'Eurobarometer is a large-scale, European cross-national, longitudinal survey research programme on attitudes, values and beliefs regarding a wide range of topics in the socio-cultural and socio-political domain on behalf of the European Commission' (Eurobarometer 2009).

11 E.g. The Wales Gene Park 'Harnessing Genetics to advance Research, Healthcare, Education and Innovation' http://www.wgp.cf.ac.uk/ (accessed 2 April 2009).

12 E.g. EMBOSS (Molecular biology), CTSim (Computed Tomography Simulator), DINO (realtime 3D visualization program for structural biology data), Genpak (manipulating DNA/RNA/protein sequences), NAMD (molecular dynamics simulation), Protein Explorer (3D molecular viewer), Ribbons (protein crystallography analysis). http://www.linux.org/apps/all/Scientific/Biology.html (accessed 8 Mar 2009).

13 Informed consent procedures have come under more sustained ethical scrutiny since the disastrous TGN1412 pharmaco trial in London in March 2006 (Alexander 2006c).

14 'The EMEA must authorise medicinal products derived from biotechnology and other high-technology processes, and medicines for certain diseases. The evaluation of evidence is delegated to regulatory agencies of Member States, including MHRA, but the concerns of all Member States are taken into account' (MHRA 2008).

> 'Before a clinical trial can be granted in the UK for a new drug, the manufacturer must obtain clinical trial authorisation (CTA) from the Medicine Healthcare Regulatory Authority (MHRA). Before a clinical trial can be authorised, the manufacturer must submit an application with supporting medical and scientific data to the MHRA. They must also obtain a positive opinion from an Ethics Committee, which is independent of the drug industry established and funded by the NHS. The supporting data partly consists of laboratory and animal testing and tests for toxicity. This data is then reviewed by the MHRA to determine whether the drug is scientifically valid and properly researched pre-clinical trial.'
>
> (Alexander 2006a).

15 'NICE has to make both scientific and social value judgments when appraising health technologies and developing clinical guidelines for the NHS. Beyond a certain threshold of production costs, a drug will be rejected by NICE. The NICE Chair and previous vice chair explain the rationale behind the decisions' (Rawlins and Culyer 2004).

16 Slogan; 'For a Better World Economy' (OECD 2005).

17 Advertising a report due out in 2007 for which no document seems to have been produced formally (OECD 2009a). See also OECD (2009b).

18 Ibid.

19 'Glivec is the medicine for chronic myeloid Leukemia (CML) and produced by Novartis. It has become famous in Korea. Its efficiency isn't the only reason for that fame. CML patients in Korea cannot get the medicine' (Jinbo 2003).

5 Genetic testing and screening

1 The publicly funded medical genetics information resource (www.genetests.org) provides a searchable database of genetically testable diseases. Tests to identify 1741 diseases were being developed by 566 clinics in June 2009.

2 How different genetic diseases differ in their transmission patterns:

- autosomal, dominant and recessive
- X-linked (X chromosome: the condition only manifests in males)
- balanced chromosomal translocations
- chromosomal abnormalities
- spontaneous mutations
- Pre-symptomatic or predictive testing is offered to asymptomatic individuals (usually) with a family history of a genetic disorder and a potential risk of eventually developing the disorder (cf. NIH 2004).

Testing for carrier status identifies usually asymptomatic individuals who have a gene mutation for an autosomal recessive, X-linked recessive or chromosomal disorder. The carrier will not usually develop the condition.

3 See Leehey *et al.* (2003) who investigate how 'carriers' of Fragile X (a single-gene inherited mental retardation condition) may not be entirely asymptomatic.

4 The HGC press release launching this said 'Should we build up a genetic profile of every newborn baby? Would it be useful? Would it be right? Could the NHS afford it?'

5 The saviour sibling issue has entered popular culture in the form of the 2009 film 'My Sister's Keeper' http://www.imdb.com/title/tt1078588/ (accessed 22 May 2009).
6 A *You and Yours* BBC Radio 4 phone-in, 11 November 2003 was held on the subject of PGD gender selection of embryos for medical and non-medical purposes.
7 A workshop on 'designer babies' was organised by Human Genetics Alert in late 2003, London, attended by Bill McKibben amongst others. See also McKibben (2003).
8 Nobel laureate Sir John Sulston speaking at an HGC open plenary session, September 2003, Cardiff.
9 See, for example, Celera's 'molecular diagnostic products that are used by hospitals and other clinical laboratories to detect, characterize, monitor and select treatment for disease', https://www.celera.com/celera/product_pipeline accessed 22 May 2009.
10 https://www.23andme.com/howitworks/ (accessed 27 April 2009).
11 Ibid.
12 See terms and conditions of use https://www.23andme.com/about/tos/ (accessed 4 November 2009).
13 Description of what services are and are not: https://www.23andme.com/about/tos/ (accessed 4 November 2009).
14 https://www.23andme.com/health/all/ (accessed 27 April 2009).

6 Genetic exceptionalism, health, identity and citizenship

1 25th anniversary edition reprinted in 2000.
2 Gene 'switches off cancer' (includes critical appraisal of newspaper reports) (NHS 2009).
3 Notes taken by the author during participant observation.
4 See ISB (2008).
5 'African Ancestry is the only company that traces your ancestry back to a specific present-day African country of origin and often to a specific African ethnic group when African ancestry is found.'(African Ancestry 2009a, b; Schramm 2007).
6 HFEA favours altruistic egg donation for cloning research (PHG 2006).
7 E.g. considerations suggested by the UK government about responsibilities to care for oneself in certain ways in order fully to access the health care system. (Prime Minister's Strategy Unit 2004; Fitzpatrick 2001).
8 'The position of the American College of Occupational and Environmental Medicine is that genetic screening is not conceptually different from other types of medical testing or screening' (ACOEM 2005).

7 Informed consent, individual choice

1 'Where screening is aimed solely at providing information to allow the person being screened to make an 'informed choice' (eg. Down's syndrome, cystic fibrosis carrier screening), there must be evidence from high quality trials that the testaccurately measures risk' (NSC 2005).
2 This document was cited in a House of Lords debate, March 2010 http://www.publications.parliament.uk/pa/d200910/ldhansrd/text/100315w0003.htm (accessed 29 April 2010).
3 http://en.wikipedia.org/wiki/Libertarian (accessed 18 June 2009).
4 In March 2004, Sense About Science and the British Endocrine Societies organised a public meeting at the Brighton Centre, Stem Cell Research: what will it do for us? http://www.senseaboutscience.org.uk/index.php/site/project/43/ accessed 26 April 2009.
5 Saviour siblings – Is it right to create a tissue-donor baby? http://www.progress.org.uk/Events/PastEventsSSL.html (accessed 26 April 2009).
6 Author's notes.

8 Futures talk

1 Author's notes, taken during event.
2 Available at http:// www.hgc.gov.uk (accessed 19 February 2009).
3 See, for example, http://www.jetpress.org/ http://www.betterhumans.com/ (both accessed 18 June 2009).
4 *Genomics, Nanotechnology and the Myth of Human Performance Enhancement' Hosted by ETC Group and Dag Hammarskjold Foundation World Social Forum 29 Jan 2005.* Text circulated via email list accessed by the author at the time.
5 *New Scientist* (2005a). Though some subsequent reports focused on medical breast reconstruction after e.g. cancer surgery; the majority of press reports emphasised the potential for cosmetic breast 'enhancement' applications.

Conclusion

1 http://indymedia.org.uk/en/2004/12/302727.html (accessed 13 December 2004).
2 ETC (2003) talks about 'Bits Atoms Neurones Genes'.
3 J. Craig Venter Institute, 'Synthetic Biology & Bioenergy' http://www.jcvi.org/cms/research/groups/synthetic-biology-bioenergy/ (accessed 3 June 2009).

Scientific Glossary

AIDS: Acquired Immune Deficiency Syndrome.

Alzheimer's: A progressive, familial neurodegenerative disorder resulting in memory loss.

Amniocentesis or chorionic villus sampling: Complemented with maternal blood tests and ultrasound, providing diagnostic testing for chromosomal disorders like **Down's syndrome**.

Autosomal: Describing a gene found outside the X and Y chromosomes and therefore not not sex-linked.

Balanced chromosomal translocation: A **Chromosome translocation** in which equal genetic material is exchanged resulting in no extra or missing part, or whole chromosomes.

Base-pair: Of **DNA**, a pair of chemical bases on opposing strands of a DNA double helix.

Bioinfomatics: The use of computer algorithms and sequence data to predict and locate functional **genes**. and predict the functions of the **proteins** they encode.

Biotech, bio-technology: Industry arising from use of recombinant DNA for specific industry needs e.g. insulin production.

Blastocyst: An embryo at the stage of implantation into the womb.

BSE: Bovine Spongiform Encephalopathy.

Carrier status: Whether a genetic descendant is a carrier of a genetically inherited disease.

Chimera: An organism which has more than one genetically distinct populations of cells. e.g. Sheep & goat chimera.

CF: Cystic Fibrosis. A genetic disease causing lung dysfunction.

Chromosomal abnormalities: Chromosomal deletions and repetitions or the presence of additional chromosomes.

Chromosomal translocation, deletion: Form of mutation in which a part of one chromosome is attached to another (translocation) or missing entirely (deletion).

Chromosome: Organisational unit of DNA, comprising: histones, DNA and other organisational and functional proteins.

Chronic (condition, symptom): Long-lasting or incurable condition.

Clone: Genetically identical organism or cell population.

Cloning therapeutic, reproductive (*see also* **CNT**): Cloning to produce therapeutically useful cell lines, or as the basis of cloning organisms e.g. Dolly the sheep, and potentially, humans.

CNT/SCNT: (Somatic) Cell Nuclear Transfer. A technique in which a nucleus from another cell is introduced into an empty egg-cell; this can be therapeutic or reproductive (**germline cloning**).

Coding: Refers to the three letter base-pair coding of a protein by a gene; code in which DNA sequences represent amino acids in a protein.

Converging technologies: For example the convergence of technologies in the **B.A.N.G** (**B**its **A**toms **N**eurons and **G**enes) laboratory, aiming to manipulate atoms, genes and neurons (*see also* **Nanobiotech**).

Curative: A treatment that will restore the patients health or cure an illness.

Diagnostic testing: Genetic testing which will give a diagnosis for an individual at risk of carrying a genetic disease, r.g. **chorionic villus sampling**.

Diploid: Having in humans the full 46 Chromosomes.

Down's syndrome: A genetic disorder in which carriers have an extra – whole or part of chromosome 21.

DNA: Deoxyribonucleic acid, the principle biological molecule of heredity.

DNA profile: A series of markers used for DNA fingerprinting and identification of individuals.

Dysmorphology: The study of abnormal (genetic) forms.

Embryo: In humans the stage after fertilization and up to 8 weeks; after which it is known as a foetus.

Epidemiology: The study of cause and distribution of disease.

Familial hypercholesterolemia (FH): A genetically inherited disorder characterised by high cholesterol often leading to early onset cardiovascular disease.

FMD: Foot and Mouth Disease.

Gene: The sequence of DNA which codes for one protein chain.

Gene expression: The production of a protein from its encoding gene.

Gene sequences: The complete **base-pair** sequence of a gene such as those produced during the **H**uman **G**ernome **P**roject.

Gene therapy: A therapy involving the reintroduction using **GM viruses** of functional genes in place of a host's faulty ones in an attempt to ameliorate or cure a genetic disease.

Genetic: Relating to inheritance or genes.

Geneticisation: Where genetics can be seen to be influencing other sciences e.g. medicine.

Genetic Markers: A gene or sequence of DNA that may be used to track the inheritance patterns or isolate a gene.

Genetic mutation: A change at the DNA level of an organism or gene.

Genetics: The study of genes, inheritance and variation. From the Greek 'genesis' for origin.

Genetic screening: Genetic testing a group of people or a population to find the prevalence of a genetic disease.

Genetic testing: Testing to find the presence of mutations, chromosome abnormalities or specific gene sequences that increase the risk of developing a disease.

Genome: The complete DNA sequence of an organism.

Genomics: The branch of genetics that studies organisms in terms of their entire genome or genetic sequence using mapping techniques.

Genotype: An individual's genetic makeup for a particular trait. e.g. left- or right-handedness.

Genotypical expression: Appearance of an individual based on genetics.

Germ cells: Cells that give rise to sperm or egg cells.

Germline cloning: Cloning for the purpose of reproduction.

GM: Genetically modified.

GM viral vectors: Genetically Modified viral vectors, for example adenovirus used to deliver self-replicating genetic material into a host e.g. in **gene therapy**.

Haemochromotosis: A genetically inherited disorder resulting in the sequestration of iron by sufferers, leading to diabetes, cirrhosis and other complications.

Haploid: Containing Half the Chromosomes present in a full set: in humans 23 chromosomes.

Haplotype: A group of **SNP** markers inherited together useful in the investigation of genetic factors behind genetic diseases and in the basis of the HapMap project, an international project aiming to record a haplotype map of the entire human genome.

HGP: Human Genome Project.

Huntington's disease (HD): A genetically inherited dominant disorder affecting neurological functions and movement.

Hybrid embryo: An embryo in which an egg is provided from one species while the nucleus from another.

Immune (response): A bodily rejection of a tissue, chemical or organism as a result of antibodies being 'raised' against the invading substance.

Immune rejection avoidance: The prevention of immune system-based rejection of an embryo e.g. during In-vitro fertilisation.

In vitro: literally 'in glass': in laboratory conditions, a test tube.

In vivo: literally 'in life' in the cell.

Inversion: In genetics a kind of mutation in which a short sequence is reversed from its proper order.

IPR: Intellectual Property Rights

IVF: In Vitro Fertilisation.

'Junk DNA': A term used initially used to describe non-coding DNA. Now obsolete in the scientific community; these regions are now suspected to have as yet unknown functional roles in **gene expression** or regulation.

Mapping: A technique used for determining the location of genes using short lengths of DNA primers and **PCR** techniques rather than sequencing.

Mass spectrometry: Technique used in identification of chemical samples, to ascertain the mass of an atom or molecule, through sequential fragmentation and ionisation.

Markers: Sequences of DNA which are specific to an area on a chromosome and can therefore be used to probe for a given gene.

MD: Muscular Dystrophy. A grouping of inherited diseases affecting motor function.

Mitochondrial DNA: The genome of a the mitochondrion organelle which provides energy inside the cell, always passed on by the mother.

Multifactorial: Disease which is heritable in that one or more disease gene will increase risk but environmental factors will determine whether the disease manifests itself.

Mutagenesis: The purposeful generation of mutation, e.g. in the development of engineered proteins.

Mutation: In DNA deviation of one base pair from the correct sequence.

Nanobiotech: The area of biotechnology that deals specifically with nano-scale products.

Nanosome: Small, nano-scale lipid walled 'bubbles' or vesicles created artificially to deliver drugs, enzymes to their targets.

Nanotechnology: Molecular machines designed for a specific purpose on the nano-scale ($1nm = 10^{-9}$ of a metre).

Neutriceuticals: Medically active compounds or nutrients, usually isolated from foodstuffs.

Nucleotide: The monomer single letter unit of the DNA biomolecule.

Nutrigenomics: The study of the effect of nutrition on genes giving rise to genome-personalised diets for example.

Oocyte: Pre-fertilisation egg.

Orphan diseases: Diseases that have a low prevalence and as a consequence receive little attention from pharmaceutical research.

Ovarian hyperstimulation syndrome (OHSS): Complication arising from the administration of fertility drugs often given in conjunction with IVF.

PCR: Polymerase Chain Reaction, a technique used to amplify quantities of **DNA** from a small sample.

PGD: Pre implantation Genetic Diagnosis. A method of screening an embryo for genetic diseases.

Pharmacogenetics: The branch of genetics that studies the inherited variation in drug responses.

Pharmacogenomics: The use of genomic information to tailor-make drugs for a an individual.

Phenotype: The visible manifestation of a genetic trait.

Phenotypical expression: The variability in physical expression of a genetic trait or **genotype.**

Pluripotent, pluripotency: The ability of for example a stem cell to give rise to any tissue type.

PND: Pre**N**atal genetic **D**iagnosis

Polycystic kidney disease: A genetic disorder characterised by cystic kidneys resulting in swelling and reduced kidney function.

Polymorphism: More than one phenotype commonly found in a population for a given trait e.g. blue eyes, brown eyes.

Predictive Testing: For example the prediction of cardiovascular disease based on genetic information.

Primitive streak: A faint line visible in an embryo which indicates the first stages of spinal cord formation.

Prognosis: A prediction of the course of a disease.

Protein: A functionally diverse set of biological molecules, coded for by DNA and composing a chain of amino acids, e.g. haemoglobin.

Proteome: The complete protein complement of an organism.

Proteomics: The study of all **proteins** encoded for and made by any given organism's genome, the **proteome**.

Recessive: A genotype masked by another.

Recombinant DNA Technology: Genetic engineering; the cutting and manipulation of DNA molecules in the laboratory e.g. the introduction of foreign genes into an organism using a vector.

Robotics, Artificial Intelligence: For example the use of robotics and artificial intelligence in the automation of genetic engineering techniques such as **DNA sequencing** and in general use for routine **recombinant DNA technology**.

SARS: **S**evere **A**ccute **R**espitory Syndrome.

Sequencing: A technique used to determine the DNA sequence or genetic code in a sample.

Sickle cell anaemia: A genetic disorder caused by a mutation in the gene coding for haemoglobin which carries oxygen in the blood.

Single gene disorder/trait: Genetic disease caused by mutation in one gene only rather than several. Often results in easily predictable familial inheritance patterns.

SNP: Single Nucleotide Polymorphisms, a single base pair variation found in the human population used for identification in DNA fingerprinting.

Spontaneous mutations: A genetic mutation occurring naturally or by chance in the cell of an organism/individual.

Stem cells (embryonic, adult): Undifferentiated or unspecialised cells that may become one or more cell type. Embryonic stem cells are **pluripotent** whereas adult stem cells may usually only become a cell from the tissue of origin.

Susceptibility genes: Particular genotypes predisposing an individual to a genetic illness.

Syndrome: A pattern of symptoms or signs that pertain to a particular disease.

Synthetic biology: The use of genetic engineering to alter or even create new life forms.

Systems biology: A more 'holistic' study of biology in which interactions between major biological systems are investigated. e.g. gene expression and immune systems.

Tay Sachs Disease (TSD): A genetic disorder of lipid metabolism most prevalent in Jewish families.

Therapeutic (treatments): Those treatments that seek to ameliorate or cure a disease e.g. the use of stem cells in the treatment of type I diabetes.

Trait: A characteristic determined by genetics.

Transgenic: Describing a genetically modified organism (**GMO**).

Transgenics: The study and techniques used in introducing the characteristics of one organisation into another by recombinant DNA technology.

Transmission patterns: How a disease is spread e.g. the discovery of malaria transmission via mosquitoes. **Variable [gene] expression:** The variability in expression or volume of protein produced by a coding gene.

Variable penetrance: The frequency, as a percentage of a certain genotype resulting in expression of a visible **trait**.

Vector: The means by which genetic material is introduced artificially into another organism. See **gene therapy**.

Viral: of viruses.

Virus: Arguably the most primitive life-form. Comprises a shell of protein containing self-replicating genetic material consisting of either DNA or RNA.

XTP: Xenotransplantation, e.g. the transplantation of a pig heart into a human being.

X chromosome: A sex chromosome, two being carried by women and one by men.

X-linked: A disease mapped to the X chromosome, X-linked recessive disorders e.g. haemophilia being more prevalent in males.

Y chromosome: Sex-determining chromosome, coding for male characteristics e.g. development of testes.

Bibliography

ACOEM (2005) *Genetic Screening in the Workplace*, Elk Grove: ACOEM.

ACPO (2005) *DNA good practice manual*, London: ACPO.

African Ancestry (2009a) *African Ancestry benefits are unparalleled*, brochure.

——(2009b) *Discover the Paternal Roots of Your Family Tree* Brochure.

Ahteensuu, M. (2004) 'The Precautionary Principle in the Risk Management of Modern Biotechnology', *Science Studies* 17: 57–65.

Ainger, K., Chesters, G., Credland, A. *et al.* (eds) (2003) *We Are Everywhere*, London: Verso.

Aldred, M.J., Crawford, P.J.M., Savarirayan, R. *et al.* (2003) 'It's only teeth – are there limits to genetic testing?' *Clinical Genetics* 63 (5): 333–9.

Alexander, A(2006a) 'Clinical drug trials – leading clinical negligence solicitor explains', Alexander Harris press release 23 March 2006.

——(2006b) 'Too much secrecy, too many questions left unanswered' Alexander Harris press release, 6 April 2006.

——(2006c) 'Specialist drugs trial solicitor criticises MHRA report into failed drugs trial' Alexander Harris press release 25 May 2006.

Altmann, J. (2004) 'Military uses of nanotechnology: perspectives and concerns', *Security Dialogue* 35 (1): 61–79.

AMRC (2003) 'AMRC statement on human embryo and stem cell research', AMRC press release May 2003.

Anderson, I. et al (eds) (2007) *Beyond Bandaids: Exploring the Underlying Social Determinants of Aboriginal Health* 'Papers from the Social Determinants of Aboriginal Health Workshop, Adelaide, July 2004', Casuarina: CRCAH.

Angell, M. (2005) *The Truth About Drug Companies: How they deceive us and what to do about it*, New York: Random House.

AP (2005) '"Stem cell therapy" craze spreads in Russia: Despite warnings, clinics and beauty salons offer treatments', *Associated Press* 14 March 2005.

APDB (2007) Australian Plant DNA Bank Ltd *Annual Report*, Lismore: APDB.

Ashcroft, A.E. (2009) *An Introduction to Mass Spectrometry* (Handout) University of Leeds.

Barry, J. (2005) 'Resistance is Fertile: from environmental to sustainability citizenship', in Bell, D.and Dobson, A. (eds) *Environment and Citizenship,* Cambridge, MA: MIT Press.

Batt, S. (1994) *Patient No More: the politics of breast cancer*, London: Scarlet Press.

Bauer, M. (ed.) (1995) *Resistance to New Technology: Nuclear Power, Information technology and Biotechnology*, Cambridge: Cambridge University Press.

Bauer, M. and Gaskell, G. (eds) (2003) *Biotechnology: The Makings of a Global Controversy*, Cambridge: Cambridge University Press.

BBC (2001) 'Cleft palate gene found', *BBC News* 16 September 2001.

——(2004a) 'Cloning milestones', *BBC News* 12 February 2004.

——(2004b) ' "Designer babies": Relax the rules?', *BBC News* 23 July 2004.

——(2006a) 'Call for inquiry into DNA samples', *BBC News* 5 January 2006.

——(2006b) 'Juveniles' DNA recording defended', *BBC News* 21 January 2006.

——(2006c) 'Zimbabweans have "shortest lives"', *BBC News* 8 April 2006.

——(2006d) 'DNA database has 50,000 children', *BBC News* 17 May 2006.

——(2007) 'Bowel cancer risk gene pinpointed', *BBC News* 8 July 2007.

——(2008a) 'Synthetic life "advance" reported', *BBC News* 24 January 2008.

——(2008b) 'Obesity gene "affects appetite"', *BBC News* 27 July 2008.

——(2008c) 'Tories warn of obesity "excuses"', *BBC News* 27 August 2008.

——(2008d) 'Windpipe transplant breakthrough', *BBC News* 19 November 2008.

——(2008e) 'Gene "triggers unhealthy eating"', *BBC News* 11 December 2008.

BBSRC (2008) 'Public–private research partnership announces £4M of projects to improve UK diet and health', BBSRC press release, 8 August 2008.

Beck, U. (1992) *Risk society; towards a new modernity*, London: Sage Publications.

——(1995) *Ecological Politics in an Age of Risk*, Cambridge: Polity Press.

Bender, W., Hauskeller, C. and Manzei, A. (eds) (2005) *Crossing Borders: Cultural, Religious and Political Differences Concerning Stem Cell Research*, Münster: Agenda Verlag.

Bharadwaj, A. (2005) 'Cultures of embryonic stem cell research in India' in Bender, W. et al. (eds) *Crossing Borders: Cultural, Religious and Political Differences Concerning Stem Cell Research*, Münster: Agenda Verlag.

Bijker, W.E. (1987) 'The social construction of bakelite: towards a theory of invention', in Bijker, W.E., Hughes, T.P. and Pinch, T.J. (eds) *The Social Construction of Technological Systems: New Directions in the Sociology and History of Technology*, Cambridge, MA: MIT Press.

Birch, K. (2006) 'The neoliberal underpinnings of the bioeconomy: the ideological discourses and practices of economic competitiveness', *Genomics, Society and Policy*, 2 (3): 1-15.

BIS (ca. 2009) 'The pharmaceutical sector in the UK', Dept of Business, Innovation and Skills handout.

Blair, A. 'Our Nation's Future', speech delivered at the Royal Society in Oxford, 3 November 2006.

——(2007) 'Speech at Blenheim Palace', delivered 1 October 2007.

Blaxter, M. (2004) *Health and Lifestyles*, London: Routledge.

Bloomberg (2008) 'Supergene labs design microbes to change sun to fuel, eat waste', *Bloomberg* 9 January 2008.

BMJ (2006) 'International consumer group slates drug marketing practices' *British Medical Journal*, 333: 14.

——(2007) 'Should genetic information be disclosed to insurers?' *BMJ* 334: 1196–7.

Boddington, P. and Clarke, A. (2004) 'It's only teeth – limits to genetic testing? A response to Aldred, Crawford, Savarirayan, and Savulescu', *Clinical Genetics* 66: 562–4.

Boddington, P. and Gregory, M. (2008) 'Communicating genetic information within the family:enriching the debate through the notion of integrity' *Medicine, Health Care and Philosophy* 11 (4): 445–54.

Boddington, P. and Hogben, S. (2006a) 'Working up policy: the use of specific disease exemplars in formulating general principles governing childhood genetic testing', *Health Care Analysis* 14 (1): 1–13.

——(2006b) 'The rhetorical construction of ethical positions:policy recommendations for non-therapeutic genetic testing in childhood', *Communication and Medicine* 3 (2): 135–46.

Borry, P., Stultiens, L., Nys, H. *et al.* (2006) 'Presymptomatic and predictive genetic testing in minors: a systematic review of guidelines and position papers', *Clinical Genetics* 70 (5): 374–81.

Borry, P., Goffin, T., Nys, H. *et al.* (2008) 'Predictive genetic testing in minors for adult-onset genetic diseases', *Mount Sinai Journal of Medicine* 75 (3): 287–96.

Bowring, F. (2003) *Science, Seeds and Cyborgs: Biotechnology and the Appropriation of Life*, London: Verso.

Bristol (2008) 'Adult stem cell breakthrough', University of Bristol press release 19 November 2008.

Brown, N. and Michael, M. (2003) 'A sociology of expectations: retrospecting pro-spects and prospecting retro-spects', *Technology Analysis and Strategic Development* 15 (1): 3–18.

Brown, P. and Zavestoski, S. (2004) 'Social movements in health: an introduction', *Sociology of Health and Illness* 26 (6): 679–94.

Bryan, E. (2007) *Singing the life; the story of a family in the shadows of cancer*, London: Vermilion.

Bucchi, M. (2004) 'Can genetics help us rethink communication? Public communica-tion of Science as a "double helix"' *New Genetics and Society* 23: 3.

Buckley, F. and Buckley, S.J. (2008) 'Wrongful deaths and rightful lives – screening for Down syndrome', *Down Syndrome Research and Practice* 12 (2): 79–86.

Burnham (2009) 'The Research of Professor Evan Snyder into Cystic Fibrosis', (Advisory), La Jolla: Burnham Institute for Medical Research.

Consumers Association (2008) 'Which? warns consumers against costly genetic tests', Consumers' Association press release, 7 July 2009.

Cabinet Office (2007) *Effective Consultation*, London: Cabinet Office.

——(2008) *Code of Practice on Consultation*, London: Cabinet Office.

Cardiff (2006) 'BBC Documentary explores University Research', Cardiff University press release 21 September 2006.

Carroll, W. and Ratner, R. (1996) 'Master framing and cross-movement metworking in contemporary social movements', *Sociological Quarterly* 37 (4): 601–25.

CEC (2001) 'Proposal for a decision of the European Parliament and the Council concerning the multiannual framework programme 2002–6 of the European Community for Research, Technological Development and Demonstration', *OJ* 21 February 2001 COM (2001) 94.

——(2002) *Life Sciences and biotechnology: A strategy for Europe*, Brussels: European Commission.

——(2004) 'Directive 2004/23/EC on setting standards of quality and safety for the donation, procurement, testing, processing, preservation, storage and distribution of human tissues and cells', *OJ* 7 April 2004.

——(2007a) *Budget breakdown of the Seventh Framework Programme of the European Community* [Leaflet] Brussels: European Commission

——(2007b) *FP7 in Brief* (Leaflet) Luxembourg: European Commission.

Celera (2008) *Celera Corporation Annual Report*, Alameda, CA: Celera Corporation.

Chadwick, R. (2005) 'HUGO Ethics Committee: ten years on', *SCRIPTed* 2 (2): 134–5.

Chadwick, R., Have, H., Husted, J. *et al.* (1998) 'Genetic screening and ethics: European perspectives', *Journal of Medicine and Philosophy* 23 (3): 255–73.

Chan, C.K. and de Wildt, G. (2007) *Developing Countries, Donor Leverage, and Access to Bird Flu Vaccines*, New York: United Nations (DESA).

Chesters, G. and Welsh, I. (2006) *Complexity and Social Movements: Protest at the Edge of Chaos*, London: Routledge.

Christiani, D., Ashfari, C., Balbus, J. *et al.* (2007) *Applications of Toxicogenomic Technologies to Predictive Toxicology and Risk Assessment*, Washington. DC: National Academies Press http://books.nap.edu/catalog.php?record_id=12037

Clarke, A. (ed.) (1998) *The Genetic Testing of Children*, Oxford: Bios Scientific Publishers.

Clinton and Blair (2000) 'Joint Statement – President Clinton and Prime Minister Blair', White House press release 14 March.

Collins, H.M. and Evans, R. (2002) 'The third wave of science studies', *Social Studies of Science* 32 (2): 235–96.

Computer Weekly (2008) 'Police to be allowed searches of national database of NHS patient records', 28 February 2008.

Consumers International (2006) *Branding the Cure*, London: Consumers International.

CORE (ca. 2005) 'About CORE' http://www.corethics.org/index.php?c=a (accessed 26 May 2009).

Corporate Watch (2005a) 'Nanotechnology: What it is and how corporations are using it' *Corporate Technologies* 1.

——(2005b) 'How many anti-nano Angels can dance on the head of a pin?' *Corporate Watch Newsletter* 22: 8.

——(2007) *Nanomaterials: Undersized, Unregulated and Already Here*, London: Corporate Watch.

——(2009) *Nestlé SA* http://www.corporatewatch.org.uk/?lid=240

Corrigan, O. (2003) 'Empty Ethics: The problem with informed consent', *Sociology of Health and Illness* 25 (3): 768–92.

Coviello, D.A., Brambati, B., Tului, L. *et al.* (2004) 'Pre First-trimester prenatal screening for the common 35delG GJB2 mutation causing prelingual deafness', *Prenatal Diagnosis* 24 (8): 631–4.

Cummins, J. (ca. 2008) 'Cauliflower mosaic virus recombination, when and where?' *Third World Network* http://www.twnside.org.sg/title/mosaic-cn.htm (accessed 15 February 2009).

Custer, N.V. (2004) *Protein Synthesis* http://www.contexo.info/DNA_Basics/Protein_synthesis.htm (accessed 8 June 2009).

Cutter, A.M. (ed.) (2006) 'Special Issue – Genomics and Criminal Justice', *Genomics, Society and Policy,* 2 (1).

DAA (2000) 'Opinion: the disabling story of gene therapy', *Disability* Tribune, February. http://web.archive.org/web/20060518175427/www.daa.org.uk/e tribune%5ce 2000 02htm

Daar, A.S. and Khitamy, A. (2001) 'Islamic bioethics', *Canadian Medical Association Journal*, 9 January, 164 (1).

Daily Mail (2009) 'My Breasts Could Kill Me', *Daily Mail* 6 July 2009.

Dawkins, R. (1976) *The Selfish Gene*, Oxford: Oxford University Press.

Davey Smith, G. and Ebrahim, S. (2005) 'What can mendelian randomisation tell us about modifiable behavioural and environmental exposures? *British Medical Journal* 330, 7 May, 1076–9.

Davey-Smith, G., Ebrahim, S., Lewis, S. *et al.* (2005) 'Genetic epidemiology and public health: hope, hype, and future prospects', The Lancet, 366 (9495): 1484–98.

DCA (1998) *Data Protection Act*, London: Dept for Constitutional Affairs.

deCODE (2007) *deCODE genetics, Inc Annual Report*, Reykjavik: decode.

Defra (2002) *Defra's Horizon Scanning Strategy for Science*, London: Defra.

Deleuze, G. and Guattari, F. (1987) *A thousand plateaus: Capitalism and schizophrenia*, Minneapolis: University of Minnesota Press.

Dept for Work and Pensions (2009) *Households Below Average Income*, London: The Stationery Office.

Dept of Health (2003) *Our inheritance, our future: realising the potential of genetics in the NHS*, London: The Stationery Office.

——(2004a) *The Medicines for Human Use (Clinical Trials) Regulations 2004*, Statutory Instrument 2004/1031.

——(2004b) *Human Tissue Act 2004*, London: The Stationery Office.

——(2008a) *End of Life Care Strategy*, London: The Stationery Office.

——(2008b) *The potential impact of an opt out system for organ donation in the UK: an independent report from the Organ Donation Taskforce*, London: The Stationery Office.

——(2008c) *Human Fertilisation and Embryology Act 2008*, London: The Stationery Office.

Dept of Health and ABI (2005) *Concordat and moratorium on genetics and insurance.* London: Dept of Health.

Di Chiro, G. (2004a) 'Local actions, global visions: remaking environmental expertise', in Eglash, R., Croissant, J., Di Chiro, G., *et al.* (eds) *Appropriating Technology: Vernacular Science and Social Power,* Minneapolis: University of Minnesota Press.

——(2004b) 'Producing "roundup ready(r)" communities? Human genome research and environmental justice policy', in Stein, R. (ed.) *New Perspectives on Environmental Justice: Gender, Sexuality, and Activism,* New Brunswick: Rutgers University Press.

——(2007) 'Indigenous peoples and biocolonialism: Defining the "science of environmental justice" in the century of the gene', in Sandler, R. and Pezzullo, P. (eds) *Environmental Justice and environmentalism: the social justice challenge to the environmental movement,* Cambridge, MA: MIT Press.

——(2008) 'Seeking the new biological fix? Public health genetics and environmental justice policy', in Molfino, F. and Zucco, F. (eds) *Women in Biotechnology: Creating Interfaces,* New York: Springer.

Diani, M. (1992) 'Analysing Social Movement Networks', in Diani, M. and Eyerman, R. (eds) *Studying Collective Action,* London: Sage.

Dickenson, D. (2002) 'Commodification of human tissue: implications for feminist and development ethics', *Developing World Bioethics*, 2 (1): 62.

——(2007) *Property in the body: feminist perspectives*, Cambridge: Cambridge University Press.

Dobson, A. (2003) *Citizenship and the Environment*, Oxford: Oxford University Press.

——(2006) 'Ecological citizenship: a defence', *Environmental Politics* 15 (3): 447–51.

Doherty, B., Plows, A. and Wall, D. (2003) 'The preferred way of doing things: The British direct action novement', *Parliamentary Affairs* 56: 669–86.

——(2007) 'Environmental direct action in Manchester, Oxford and North Wales: a protest event analysis', *Environmental Politics* 16 (5): 805–25.

Dryzek, J. S. (2000) *Deliberative Democracy and Beyond: Liberals, Critics, Contestations*, Oxford: Oxford University Press.

DTI (2002) *New Dimensions for Manufacturing: A UK Strategy for Nanotechnology*, London: DTI.

ECHR (2008) 'Grand Chamber Judgement S. and Marper v. The United Kingdom', ECHR press release 4 December 2008.

EGE (2000) *Ethical aspects of human stem cell research and use*, Brussels: European Commission.

——(2005) *General Report on the Activities of the European Group on Ethics in Science and New Technologies to the European Commission 2000–2005*, Luxembourg: European Communities.

EGP (1997) *Environmental Genome Project*, Research Triangle Park: NIEHS.

Einsiedel, E., Allum, N., Bauer, M. *et al.* (2003) 'Brave new sheep – the clone named Dolly', in Bauer, M. and Gaskell, G. (eds) *Biotechnology: The Makings of a Global Controversy,* Cambridge: Cambridge University Press.

E-Petition (2007) 'Stop DNA by Stealth', (Petition) http://petitions.pm.gov.uk/StopDNAbystealth/ (accessed 16 May 2007).

Epstein, S. (2004) 'Bodily differences and collective identities: the politics of gender and race in biomedical research in the United States', *Body & Society* 10 (2–3): 183–203.

——(2007) *Inclusion. The Politics of Difference in Medical Research*, Chicago: University of Chicago Press.

Eriksson, L. (2004) 'When Scientists Fight', *Science & Public Affairs,* June, 25.

Eschle, C. (2001) 'Globalizing civil society? Social movements and the challenge of global politics from below', in Hamel, P., Lustiger-Thaler, H., Pieterse, J. *et al.* (eds) *Globalization and Social Movements,* Basingstoke: Palgrave Macmillan.

Eschle, C. and Stammers, N. (2005) 'Social movements and global activism', in De Yong, W., Shaw, M. and Stammers, N. (eds) *Global Activism, Global Media,* London: Pluto Press, pp. 50–67.

ESSFN (2005) *Framework Programme 7: Towards a real partnership with society*, European Science Social Forum Network http://www.scienceforthepeople.com/index.php?name=News&file=article& sid = 59

ETC Group (2003) *The Big Down: Atomtech – Technologies Converging at the Nanoscale*, Ottawa: ETC Group.

——(2004) 'White papers, red flags, green goo, grey goo (and red herrings)', *ETC Group Communiqué* Issue 85.

——(2008a) *Direct-to-Consumer DNA Testing and the Myth of Personalized Medicine: Spit Kits, SNP Chips and Human Genomics*, Ottawa: ETC Group.

——(2008b) 'Who owns nature? Corporate power and the final frontier in the commodification of life', *ETC Group Communiqué* Issue 100.

——(2009) *The Issues* http://www.etcgroup.org/en/issues/ (accessed 29 May 2009).

Ethox (2005) 'Governing genetic databases' (Mission statement).

Eurobarometer (2009) *European cross-national, longitudinal survey*, Brussels: CEC.

Evans, R and Plows, A. (2007) 'Listening without prejudice? Re-discovering the value of the disinterested citizen', Social Studies of Science 37 (6): 827–53.

Evans, R., Welsh, I. and Plows, A. (2006) 'Towards an anatomy of public engagement with medical genetics: strange bedfellows and usual suspects', in Atkinson, P., Glasner, P. and Greenslade, H.(eds) *New Genetics, New Identities,* London: Routledge.

——(2008) 'Just around the corner: rhetorics of progress and promise in genetic research', *Public Understanding of Science* 18 (1): 43–59.

Evans, W.E. and Relling, M. (1999) 'Pharmacogenomics: translating functional genomics into rational therapeutics', *Science* 286: 487–91.

Featherstone, K., Atkinson, P., Bharadwaj, A. *et al.* (2006) *Risky relations: family, kinship and the new genetics*, Oxford: Berg.

Financial Times (2009) 'Are medical surveys good for our health?' 7 February.

Fischer, F. (2000) *Citizens, Experts, and the Environment: The Politics of Local Knowledge*, Durham, NC: Duke University Press.

Fitzpatrick, M. (2001) *The Tyranny of Health: Doctors and the Regulation of Lifestyle*, London: Routledge.

Ford, L.H. (2003) 'Challenging global environmental governance: social movement agency and global civil society', *Global Environmental Politics*, 3 (2): 120–34.

Foucault, M. (2003) 'The birth of biopolitics', in Rabinow, P. and Rose, N. (eds) *The Essential Foucault: Selections From the Essential Works of Foucault 1954–1984*, New York: New Press.

Franklin, S. (2007) *Dolly Mixtures: the remaking of genealogy*, Durham, NC: Duke University Press.

——(2008) 'Embryo transfer: a view from the United Kingdom', in Molfino, F. and Zucco, F. (eds) *Women in Biotechnology: Creating Interfaces,* New York: Springer.

Franklin, S. and Roberts, C. (2006) *Born and Made: An Ethnography of Preimplantation Genetic Diagnosis*, Princeton, NJ: Princeton University Press.

Fukuyama, F. (2002) *Our Posthuman Future: Consequences of the Biotechnology Revolution*, New York: Farrar, Straus, and Giroux.

Furedi, Frank (2002) *Culture of fear: risk-taking and the morality of low expectation*, London: Continuum.

Gardner, P. (2003) 'Distorted packaging: marketing depression as illness, drugs as cure', *Journal of Medical Humanities* 24: 105–30.

Gelsinger, P. (2008) 'A comment from Paul Gelsinger on gene therapy and informed consent', *American Journal of Bioethics blog.bioethics.net* http://blog.bioethics.net/2008/01/a-comment-from-paul-gelsinger-on-gene-therapy-and/ accessed 15 February 2009.

GeneWatch (2000) *Privatising Knowledge, Patenting Genes: The Race to Control Genetic Information* #Briefing 11, Buxton: GeneWatch.

——(2002a) *Human Genetics and Health*, Buxton: GeneWatch.

——(2002b) *Genetically Modified and Cloned Animals. All in a Good Cause?* Buxton: GeneWatch.

——(2004) 'Bar-Coding Babies: Good for Health?' *GeneWatch* #Briefing 27, 1 August 2004, Buxton: GeneWatch.

——(2004) *Genetic Tests and Health; the Case for Regulation* #Briefing 28, Buxton: GeneWatch.

——(2005) *The Police National DNA Database: Human Rights and Privacy*, Buxton: GeneWatch.

——(2006a) 'NDNAD facts and figures' http://www.genewatch.org/sub.shtml?als[cid]=539481 (accessed 16 May 2007).

——(2006b) *Using the police National DNA Database – under adequate control?* Buxton: GeneWatch.

——(2007) 'Regulation needed to prevent human genome from becoming massive marketing scam', GeneWatch press release 29 October 2007.

——(2008) *Modernising police powers* http://www.genewatch.org/sub/shtml?als[cid]=551990 (accessed 16 May 2007).

——(2009a) GeneWatch UK believes that genetic horoscopes are a dangerous myth' http://www.genewatch.org/sub.shtml?als%5Bcid%5D=532295 (accessed 10 February 2009).

——(2009b) *Is 'early health' good health? The implications of genomic data-mining in the NHS*, Buxton: GeneWatch.

——(2009c) *Examples of genes and common diseases*, Buxton: GeneWatch.

——(2009d) 'A brief legal history of the NDNAD' http://www.genewatch.org/sub.shtml?als[cid]=537968 (accessed 16 May 2007).

GeneWatch, ARCH, Liberty(2007) *NDNAD: proposed expansions of powers*, Buxton: GeneWatch.

Genographic Project (2008) 'Your genetic journey' (Brochure).

GHR (2008) 'What are the CYP genes?' *Genetics Home Reference,* Bethesda: U.S. National Library of Medicine.

Gibbons, S.M.C., Kaye, J., Smart, A. *et al.* (2007) 'Governing genetic databases: challenges facing research regulation and practice'. *Journal of Law and Society* 34 (2): 163-89.

Gibson, A.G. (1933) *The Physician's Art*, Oxford: The Clarendon Press.

Glasner, P. and Rothman, H. (2004) *Splicing Life? The New Genetics and society*, Aldershot: Ashgate.

Goffman, E. (1974) *Frame analysis: An essay on the organization of experience,*New York: Harper & Row.

Goodman, E. and Adler, N. (2007) 'The biology of social justice: linking social inequalities and health in adolescence', in Wainryb, C., Smetana, J. and Elliot Turiel, T.(eds) *Social Development, Social Inequalities, and Social Justice*, London: Psychology Press.

Granovetter, M.S. (1973) 'The strength of weak ties', *American Journal of Sociology* 78 (6): 1360–80.

Green Action (2004) *Technology, Politics, and Democracy*, Belfast: Green Action.

Greenpeace (2005) 'Nano jury "verdict" calls for more public say and clarity on nanotechnology', Greenpeace press release 21 September 2005.

Grove-White, R., Macnaghten, P. and Wynne, B. (2000), *Wising Up: The public and new technologies*, Lancaster: IEPPP.

Guardian (2000) 'DNA sequences (partial and complete gene sequences) which have been recorded in patents from 40 patent authorities worldwide', 8 March 2000.

——(2002) 'One man and his worm', 9 October 2002.

——(2006) 'Controversial conceptions', 9 May 2006.

——(2008a) 'Early humans helped to develop with "junk" DNA', 5 September 2008.

——(2008b) 'Hannah's Choice', 12 November 2008.

——(2008c) 'Father tells inquest of son's dying moments', 11 December 2008.

——(2009a) 'She may never get breast cancer – but girl's birth raises new doubts over designer babies', 10 January 2009.

——(2009b) '"Neanderthals" genetic code reconstructed by researchers'. 13 February 2009.

Habermas, J. (1981) *The theory of communicative action*, Boston: Beacon Press.

——(1987) *The theory of communicative action: A critique of functionalist reason*, vol. 2, *Lifeworld and System*, London: Polity Press.

——(2003) *The Future of Human Nature*, Oxford: Polity Press.

Hamilton, W.D. (1964). 'The genetical evolution of social behavior', *Journal of Theoretical Biology* 7 (1): 1–52.

Hammersley, M. (ed.) (1993) *Social Research: Philosophy, Politics and Practice*, London: Sage.

Hansard (2002) *HL debate Stem Cell Research, Hansard* 5 December 2002: col. 1311.

——(2004) 'Human fertilisation and embryology act donor identity', *Hansard* 21 January 2004: col. 60WS.

——(2006a) 'DNA database volunteers', *Hansard* 16 January 2006: col. 1094W.

——(2006b) 'DNA database under 18', *Hansard* 2 May 2006: col. 1409W.

——(2007a) 'HL debate stem cell research', *Hansard* 3 May 2007: col. 1163.

——(2007b) 'Genetics: databases', *Hansard* 10 May 2007: col. 427W.

——(2008) 'Human fertilisation and embryology bill debate', *Hansard* 12 May 2008: col. 1063.

Haran, J. and O'Riordan, K. (2006) 'Women, feminism and human cloning: recirculating concerns and critiques', *Feminist Media Studies* 6(2): 217–22.

Haran, J., Kitzinger, J., McNeil, M. and O'Riordan, K. (2007) *Human Cloning in the Media: From Science Fiction to Science Practice*, London: Routledge.

Haraway, D. (1991) 'A cyborg manifesto: science, technology, and socialist-feminism in the late twentieth century', in *Simians, Cyborgs and Women: The Reinvention of Nature*, New York, London: Routledge.

Harcourt, W. (2008) 'Heading blithely down the garden path? Some entry points into current debates on women and biotechnologies', in Molfino, F. and Zucco, F. (eds) *Women in Biotechnology: Creating Interfaces*, New York: Springer.

Harris, J. (2005) 'Scientific research is a moral duty', *Journal of Medical Ethics* 31: 242–8.

Harry, D., Howard, S. and Shelton, B.(2000) *Indigenous Peoples, Genes and Genetics. What Indigenous People Should Know About Biocolonialism*, Nixon, NV: Indigenous Peoples Council on Biocolonialism.

Hayward, T. (2005) *Constitutional Environmental Rights*, Oxford: Oxford University Press.

——(2006) 'Ecological citizenship: justice, rights and the virtue of resourcefulness', *Environmental Politics* 15(3): 435–46.

HC 2005 *House of Commons Science and Technology Committee: Forensic Science on Trial*, London: The Stationery Office.

——(2007) *House of Commons Science and Technology Committee: Fifth Report*, London: The Stationery Office.

HoC Library (2009) *Retention of fingerprint and DNA data*, London: HoC Library.

HealthDataRights (2009) 'Thought-leaders unite to release declaration of health data rights', Health Data Rights press release 22 June 2009.

Herring, J. (2006) *Medical Law and Ethics*, Oxford: Oxford University Press.

HFEA (2001) 'HFEA to allow tissue typing in conjunction with preimplantation genetic diagnosis' HFEA Press Release 13 Dec 2001.

——(2003) 'Court of Appeal allows tissue typing for human embryos under strict conditions', HFEA press release 12 March 2009.

——(2006) *Donating eggs for research: safeguarding donors*, London: HFEA.

——(2007) 'Statement on donating eggs for research', HFEA press release 21 February 2007.

HGA (2000) *The regulation of pre-implantation genetic diagnosis*, London: HGA.

——(2003) 'Why it is wrong to select embryos to be tissue donors' (Commentary) press release 20 June.

HGC and NSC (2005) *Profiling the Newborn*, London: Human Genetics Commission.

HGC (2002) *Inside Information: Balancing Interests in the Use of Genetic Data*, London: Human Genetics Commission.

——(2003) *Direct Genetic Testing*, London: Human Genetics Commission.

——(2004) *Choosing the future:genetics and reproductive decision making*, London: Human Genetics Commission.

——(2007) *Joint committee on the Human Tissue and Embryos (Draft) Bill – First Report*, HC 630-I, HL Paper 169-I 1 August 2007, London: The Stationery Office.

——(2009) *Genomic Medicine Inquiry*, London: The Stationery Office.

Ho, M-W. (2003) *Living With the Fluid Genome*, London: Institute of Science and Society.

Hogben, S. and Boddington, P. (2005) 'Policy recommendations for carrier testing and predictive testing in childhood: a distinction that makes a real difference', *Journal of Genetic Counselling* 14 (4): 271–82.

Home Office (2006) *DNA Expansion Programme 2000–2005: Reporting achievement*, London: Home Office.

——(2007a) *Modernising Police Powers: Review of the Police and Criminal Evidence Act (PACE) 1984*, (March 2000) London: Home Office.

——(2007b) 'Thousands of "cold cases" to be reviewed', Home Office press release 11 September 2007.

——(2009) *Research and testing using animals*, Home Office handout.

HOOO (2006) 'Korea Herald: Seoul tightens egg/sperm donation rules', *Hands off our ovaries Newsletter*, 20 November 2006.

Hope (2004) *Medical Ethics: a Very Short Introduction*, Oxford: Oxford University Press.

Hopkins, M.M., Martin, P., Nightingale, P. *et al.* (2007) 'The myth of the biotech revolution: An assessment of technological, clinical and organisational change', *Research Policy* 36 (4): 566–89.

Horlick-Jones, T., Walls, J., Rowe, G. *et al.* (2007) *The GM Debate: Risk, Politics and Public Engagement*, London: Routledge.

Horlick-Jones, T., Walls, J. and Kitzinger, J. (2007) 'Bricolage in action: learning about, making sense of, and discussing, issues about genetically modified crops and food', *Health, Risk & Society* 9 (1): 83–103.

Howard, S. (2001) *Life, Lineage and Sustenance: Indigenous Peoples and Genetic Engineering, Threats to Food, Agriculture and the Environment*, Nixon, NV: Indigenous Peoples Council on Biocolonialism.

HUGO (2000) *Statement on Benefit-Sharing*, Vancouver: HUGO.

Hütter, G., Nowak, D., Mossner, M. *et al.* (2009) 'Long-term control of HIV by CCR5 Delta32/Delta32 stem-cell transplantation', *New England Journal of Medicine* 360 (7): 692–8.

Illich, I. (1975) *Limits to Medicine: Medical Nemesis The Appropriation of Health*, London: Marian Boyers.

Independent (1997) 'After Dolly comes Polly, the sheep with human genes', 25 July 1997.

——(2008) 'Brown wins 42-day detention vote by a whisker', 11 June 2008.

——(2009) 'Gene therapy offers hope of cure for HIV', 12 February 2009.

IPO (2009) *IPO Examination Guidelines for Patent Applications relating to Biotechnological Inventions in the Intellectual Property Office*, Newport, Gwent: IPO.

Irwin, A. (1995) *Citizen Science; A Study of People, Expertise and Sustainable Development*, London: Routledge.

Irwin, A. and Michael, M. (2003) *Science, Theory and Public Knowledge*, Maidenhead: Open University Press.

Irwin, A. and Wynne, B. (eds) (1996) *Misunderstanding Science? The Public Reconstruction of Science and Technology*, Cambridge: Cambridge University Press.

ISB (2008) *Institute for Systems Biology Annual Report 2007* Seattle: ISB.

ISESCO (2005) 'Human Genetic and Reproductive Technologies: Comparing Religious and Secular Perspectives' Seminar in 2005 Organised by The Islamic Educational Scientific & Cultural Organisation (ISESCO) and Human Genetics Alert (HGA), London.

Ishiguro, K. (2005) *Never Let Me Go*, London: Faber and Faber.

Jasanoff, S. (1990) *The fifth branch. Science advisers as policymakers*, Cambridge, MA: Harvard University Press.

——(1995) 'Product, process, or programme: three cultures and the regulation of biotechnology', in Bauer, M. (ed.) *Resistance to New Technology*, Cambridge: Cambridge University Press.

——(2005a) *Designs on Nature: Science and Democracy in Europe and the United States*, Princeton, NJ: Princeton University Press.

——(2005b) 'Science and environmental citizenship', in Dauvergne, P. (ed.) *Handbook of Global Environmental Politics*, Cheltenham: Edward Elgar.

JINBO (2003) *Struggle for Access to Glivec in South Korea* http://glivec.jinbo.net/what_en.html (accessed 29 May 2009).

KCL (2004) 'Stem cell hope for degenerative disorders'. King's College London press release 8 September 2004.

Keller, E.F. (2000) *The Century of the Gene*, Harvard: Harvard University Press.

Kerr, A. and Shakespeare, T. (2002) *Genetic Politics – From Eugenics to Genome*, Gloucester: New Clarion Press.

Kerr, A., Cunningham-Burley, S. and Amos, A.(1998a) 'The new genetics and health: mobilizing lay expertise', *A Public Understanding of Science* 7: 41–60.

——(1998b). 'Drawing the line: an analysis of lay people's discussion about the new genetics', *A Public Understanding of Science* 7: 113–33.

King's Fund (2008) *NHS spending: Local variations in priorities: an update*, London: King's Fund.

Knorr-Cetina, K. (1999) *Epistemic Cultures: How the Sciences Make Knowledge*, Cambridge, MA: Harvard University Press.

Lackner, K.J. (2002) 'From pharmacogenetics to pharmacogenomics', *Trends in Pharmacological Sciences* 23(1): 46.

Latour, B. (1993) *We Have Never Been Modern*, Cambridge, MA: Harvard University Press.

Latour, B. and Woolgar, S. (1979) *Laboratory Life: The Social Construction of Scientific Facts*, London: Sage.

Law, J. (2006) *After Method: Mess in Social Science Research*, London: Routledge.

Leehey, M., Munhoz, R., Lang, A. *et al.* (2003) ' The fragile X premutation presenting as essential tremor' *Archives of Neurology* 60: 117–21.

Levitt, M. and Tomasini, F. (2006) 'Bar-coded children: an exploration of issues around the inclusion of children on the England and Wales National DNA database', *Genomics, Society and Policy* 2 (1): 41-56.

Liberty (2008) 'Shadow Home Secretary resigns over extending pre-charge detention for terror suspects to 42 days' Liberty press release 12 June.

Lichtenstein, P., Holm, N., Verkasalo, P. *et al* (2000) 'Environmental and heritable factors in the causation of cancer – analyses of cohorts of twins from Sweden, Denmark, and Finland', *New England Journal Medicine* July, 343 (2): 78–85.

Lippman, A. (1991) 'Prenatal genetic testing and screening: constructing needs and reinforcing inequities', *American Journal of Law and Medicine* 17 (1-2): 15–50.

Lunshof, J., Chadwick, R., Vorhaus, D. *et al.* (2008) 'From genetic privacy to open consent', *Nature Reviews Genetics* May, 9: 406–11.

McAdam, D. (1986) 'Recruitment to high-risk activism: the case of Freedom Summer', *American Journal of Sociology* 92 (1): 64–90.

McConkie-Rosell, A. and DeVellis, B.M. (2000) 'Threat to parental role: a possible mechanism of altered self-concept related to carrier knowledge', *Journal of Genetic Counseling* 9 (4): 285–302.

McKibben, B. (2003) *Enough: Staying Human in an Engineered Age*, New York: Henry Holt.

Macmillan Cancer Support (2009) 'A breast cancer break through', 11 January 2009 http://www.whatnow.org.uk/blog/jan2/breast-cancer-break-through (accessed 18 June) 2009.

McMurtry, J. (1999) *The Cancer Stage of Capitalism*, London: Pluto Press.

McNally, R. and Glasner, P. (2007) *Survival of the gene? Twenty first century visions from genomics, proteomics and the new biology*, London: Routledge.

Magnus, D. and Cho, M.K. (2006) 'Issues in oocyte donation for stem cell research', *Science* 19 May 2005.

Marks, J. (2007) *'How does genomics change our understanding of society?'* Keynote speech at the Economic and Social Research Council's Genomics Network conference 'Today Answers, Tomorrow Questions', London, 25 October 2007 available as an MP3 audio file at http://www.genomicsnetwork.ac.uk/media/marksnoq&a2.mp3 (accessed 16 June 2009).

Marmot, M.G and Shipley, M.J (1996) 'Do socioeconomic differences in mortality persist after retirement? 25 Year follow up of civil servants from the first Whitehall study', *BMJ* 313: 1177–80.

Mayer, S. (2002). 'From genetic modification to nanotechnology: the dangers of "sound science"', in Gilland, T. (ed.) *Science: can we trust the experts?* London: Hodder & Stoughton.

Mayrhofer, M. and Prainsack, B. (2009), 'Being a member of the club: the transnational (self-)governance of networks of biobanks', *International Journal of Risk Assessment and Management* 12 (1): 64–81.

Melucci, A. (1996) *Challenging Codes: Collective Action in the Information Age*, Cambridge: Cambridge University Press.

MHRA (2008) *Who makes the decisions?* (Leaflet), February.

Midden, C., Boy, D., Einsiedel, E. *et al.* (2002) 'The structure of public perceptions', in Bauer, M. and Gaskell, G. (eds) *Biotechnology: The Makings of a Global Controversy,* Cambridge: Cambridge University Press.

Mies, M. and Shiva, V. (1993) *Ecofeminism*, London: Zed Books.

Miller, P. and Wilsdon, J. (eds) (2006) *Better Humans? The politics of human enhancement and life extension*, London: Demos.

Mitchell, D. (2004) *Cloud Atlas*, London: Sceptre.

Mohrenweiser, H., Wilson, D. and Jones, I. (2003) 'Challenges and complexities in estimating both the functional impact and the disease risk associated with the extensive genetic variation in human DNA repair genes', *Mutation Research/ Fundamental and Molecular Mechanisms of Mutagenesis* 526 (1): 93–125.

MRC (2005) *Research regulation and ethics*, London: MRC.

Mulkay, M. (1993) 'Rhetorics of hope and fear in the great embryo debate', *Social Studies of Science* 23 (4): 721–42.

Nahman, M. (2006) 'Materializing Israeliness: difference and mixture in transnational ova donation', *Science as Culture* 15 (3): 199–213.

Nature (2006a) 'Rise and fall', *Nature* 11 January 2006.
——(2006b) 'Health effects of egg donation may take decades to emerge', *Nature* 9 August 2006.
NBPA (2006) 'DNA breakthrough', National Black Police Association press release 16 October 2006.
NCoB (2002) *Genetics and Human Behaviour: the Ethical Context*, London: Nuffield Council on Bioethics.
——(2003) *Pharmacogenetics: Ethical Issues*, London: Nuffield Council on Bioethics.
——(2006) 'Ethical questions over police use of DNA', Nuffield CoB press release 1 November 2006.
——(2007) 'DNA of innocent people should not be kept by police', Nuffield CoB press release 18 September 2007.
NDNAD Ethics Group (2008) *1st Annual Report by the National DNA Database Ethics Group*, London: NPIA.
Nelkin, D. (1995) 'Forms of intrusion: comparing resistance to information technology and biotechnology in the USA', in Bauer, M. (ed.) *Resistance to new Technology: Nuclear Power, Information Technology and Biotechnology*, Cambridge: Cambridge University Press.
NetDoctor (ca. 2008) *Why is ADHD controversial?* http://www.netdoctor.co.uk/adhd/whyisadhdcontroversial.htm (accessed 11 February 2009).
New Scientist (2002) 'Genetic basis for lactose intolerance', 14 January 2002.
——(2005a) 'Stem cells turn into breast implants', 18 February 2005.
——(2005b) 'Will DNA profiling fuel prejudice?' 8 April 2005.
——(2006a) 'Interview: Tony Blair on science', 4 November 2006.
——(2006b) 'Catastrophic immune response may have caused drug trial horror', 17 March 2006.
——(2008) 'Junk DNA may have handed us a gripping future', 4 September 2009.
——(2008) 'Thousands volunteer to expose DNA secrets to the world', 21 October 2008.
New York Times (2009) 'A Genetics Company Fails, Its Research too Complex' (Nicholas Wade), 17 November.
Ngwena, C. and Chadwick, R. (1993) 'Genetic diagnostic information and the duty of confidentiality: ethics and law', *Medical law international* 1 (1): 73–95.
NHS (2007) 'I want to try for a baby. Should I seek genetic counselling? NHS leaflet.
——(2009) 'Gene "switches off cancer"',' *NHS News,* 2 February 2009.
——CSP (2004) 'Cervical Screening Guide', NHS leaflet.
NICE (2008) 'Antenatal care: routine care for the healthy pregnant woman', London: NICE.
Nightingale, P. and Martin, P. (2004) 'The myth of the biotechnology revolution', *Trends in Biotechnology* 22 (11): 564–9.
NIH (1990) 'Human Genome Project', NIH press release.
——(2002a) 'International consortium launches genetic variation mapping project: HapMap will help identify genetic contributions to common diseases', NIH press release October 2002.
——(2002b) 'The mouse genome and the measure of man', NIH news advisory, December 2002.
NO2ID (2008) 'Halt biometric bullying by roadside fingerprinting', NO2ID press release 27 October 2008.
Nordmann, A. (2008) 'No future for nanotechnology? Historical development vs global expansion', in Jotterand, F. (ed.) *Emerging Conceptual, Ethical and Policy Issues in Bionanotechnology*, New York: Springer.

Norsigian, J. (2005) 'Egg donation for IVF and stem cell research: time to weigh the risks to women's health', *DifferenTakes* 33, Spring.

NPIA (2007) *Annual Report for the National DNA Database 2006 – 2007*, London: National Policing Improvement Agency.

NSC (2005) *Policy Review Process*, London: National Screening Committee.

Observer (2006) 'Police DNA database "is spiralling out of control": Secret emails show private firms store genetic data from innocent victims', 16 July 2006.

——(2008) 'To save lives, we have to change attitudes to organ donation', 16 November 2008.

——(2008) 'Internet gene tests provoke alarm', 3 February 2008.

OCA (2003) 'Battle over cancer gene test U.S. company's patenting claim called "abhorrent"', *Organic Consumers Association Newsletter,* September 2003 http://www.purefood.org/Patent/010903_patent.cfm (accessed 8 March 2009).

OECD (2005) Organisation Chart, Paris: OECD.

——(2006) *Creation and Governance of Human Genetic Research Databases*, Paris: OECD.

——(2007a) *Pharmacogenetics: Opportunities and Challenges for Health Systems*, OECD handout.

——(2007b) 'The impacts of pharacogenetics on health systems', *Health Update Newsletter* 2007 (3): 16.

——(2008) *Guidelines for Human Biobanks and Genetic Research Databases*, Paris: OECD.

——(2009a) *Pharmacogenetics: Opportunities and Challenges for Health Systems*, Paris: OECD.

——(2009b) *The Bioeconomy to 2030: Designing a Policy Agenda*, Paris: OECD.

O'Riordan, K. and Haran, J. (2009) 'From reproduction to research: sourcing eggs, IVF and cloning in the UK', *Feminist Theory* 10 (2): 191–210.

PAE (2004) 'Anti eugenics action', People Against Eugenics press release 18 May 2003.

Parker, M. and Lucassen, A. (2003) 'Concern for families and individuals in clinical genetics', *Journal of Medical Ethics* 29: 70–3.

Parry, S. (2006) '(Re)constructing embryos in stem cell research: Exploring the meaning of embryos for people involved in fertility treatments', *Social Science & Medicine* 62 (2006) 2349–59.

Pears, T. (2002) *Wake up*, London: Bloomsbury.

PET (2004) 'HFEA to change its mind on "saviour siblings"?' Progress Educational Trust press release.

——(2005) 'About BioNews', *BioNews* http://www.bionews.org.uk/aboutbionews.lasso (accessed 2 September 2005).

——(2007) FIND genetic databases used by the police help them solve http://www.progress.org.uk/Events/PastEventsDDNAC.html (accessed 16 May 2007).

——(ca. 2008) *About Progress Educational Trust* http://www.progress.org.uk/About/Index.html (accessed 21 May 2009).

PHG (2006) 'HFEA favours altruistic egg donation for cloning research', Foundation for Genomics and Population Health press release 16 February 2006.

PHM (2009) *Intellectual Property and Pharmaceuticals* http://phmoz.org/wiki/index.php?title=Intellectual_Property_and_Pharmaceuticals (accessed 17 April 2009).

Pickering, S.J. and Braude, P. (2003) 'Preimplantation genetic diagnosis as a novel source of embryos for stem cell research', *Reproductive biomedicine online* (October)

7(3): 353–64 http://www.rbmonline.com/4DCGI/Article/2003/1074/RB1074.pdf (accessed 22 June 2009).

PICTF (2001) *Pharmaceutical Industry Competitiveness Task Force: Final Report,* London: The Stationery Office.

Plows, A. (2003) 'Praxis and practice: the "what, how and why" of the UK environmental direct action (EDA) movement in the 1990s', Ph.D. Bangor, University of Wales.

——(2004) 'Activist networks in the UK: mapping the build-up to the anti-globalization movement', in Carter, J. and Morland, D. (eds) *Anti-Capitalist Britain,* Gloucester: New Clarion Press.

——(2006) 'PGD, PND and the challenge of "informed choice" for feminism', *PropEur newsletter* 2, p. 4.

——(2007a) 'You've been framed! Why publics mistrust the policy process', *Genomics Network newsletter* 6: 22–3.

——(2007b) 'Regulating egg donation for research: putting the cart before the horse?' *Bionews* 22 February 2007 http://www.bionews.org.uk/commentary.lasso?storyid=3315

——(2008a) 'Social movements and ethnographic methodologies: an overview of key issues using case study examples', *Sociological Compass* August 2008.

——(2008b) 'Egg donation in the UK: tracing emergent networks of feminist engagement in relation to HFEA policy shifts in 2006', in Molfino, F. and Zucco, F. (eds) *Women in Biotechnology: Creating Interfaces,* New York: Springer.

——(2008c) 'Towards an analysis of the "success" of UK green protests'. *British Politics* (2008) 3: 92-109.

Plows, A. and Boddington, P. (2006) 'Troubles with biocitizenship?' *Genetics, Society and Policy* 2 (3): 115-35.

Plows, A. and Reinsborough, M. (2008) 'Nanobiotechnology and ethics: converging civil society discourses', in Jotterand, F. (ed.) *Emerging Conceptual, Ethical and Policy Issues in Bionanotechnology,* New York: Springer.

Plows, A., Wall, D. and Doherty, B. (2004) 'Covert repertoires: ecotage in the UK', *Social Movement Studies* 3 (2)199–219.

Plows, A., Haran, J. and O'Riordan, K. (2006) *Should scientific researchers be allowed to ask women to provide their eggs for disease research?* Cardiff: CESAGen.

Poore, C. (2007) *Disability in Twentieth-Century German Culture,* Ann Arbor: University of Michigan.

PR Watch (2003) 'From patient activism to astroturf marketing', *PR Watch* 10 (1).

Prainsack, B., Reardon, J., Hindmarsh, R. *et al.* (2008) 'Personal genomes: Misdirected precaution', *Nature* 456: 34–5.

Prime Minister's Strategy Unit (2004) *Personal Responsibility and Changing Behaviour: the state of knowledge and its implications for public policy,* London: Cabinet Office.

Primrose, S.B. and Twyman, T.M. (2006) *Principles of gene manipulation and genomics,* Oxford: Blackwell.

PSP (2004) *Public Attitudes to Stem Cell Research – establishing the UK stem cell bank,* London: People Science and Policy.

Purdue, D. (2000) *Anti-GentiX: The emergence of the Anti-GM movement,* Aldershot: Avebury.

PXE (2004) 'U.S. patent office issues first gene patent to patient advocacy group; co-inventors include non-scientist "Mom"', PXE press release 24 August 2004.

Rabinow, P. (1996) 'Artificially and enlightenment: from sociobiology to biosociality', in Rabinow, P., *Essays on the Anthropology of Reason,* Princeton, NJ: Princeton University Press.

Rahman, Q. (2008) 'Asbestos past experiences, nanoparticles future developments', in Molfino, F. and Zucco, F. (eds) *Women in Biotechnology: Creating Interfaces,* New York: Springer.

Rajan, S.K. (2006) *Biocapital: the constitution of postgenomic life,* Durham, NC: Duke University Press.

Rapp, R. (1999) *Testing Women, Testing the Fetus: The Social Impact of Amniocentesis in America,* London: Routledge.

Rawlins, M.D. and Culyer, A.J. (2004) 'National Institute for Clinical Excellence and its value judgments', *BMJ* 329 (7459): 224–7.

Register (2008) 'How to delete your DNA profile', *The Register,* 7 January 2008. http://www.theregister.co.uk/2008/01/07/delete_your_dna_profile/ (accessed 22 July 2009).

ReproKult (2005) Home Page http://www.reprokult.de/e_welcome.html (accessed 26 May 2005).

Richards, M. (2001) 'How distinctive is genetic information?' *Stud. Hist. Phil. Biol. & Biomed. Sci* 32 (4): 663–87.

Riessman, C.K. (2005) 'Exporting ethics: a narrative about narrative research in South India', *Health* 9 (4): 473–90.

Roco, M.C. and Bainbridge, W.S. (eds) (2003) *Converging Technologies for Improving Human Performance: Nanotechnology, Biotechnology, Information Technology and Cognitive Science,* Dordrecht: Kluwer.

Rose, N. (2001) 'The politics of life itself', *Theory, Culture and Society* 18 (6): 1–30.

Rose, N. and Novas, C. (2004) 'Biological citizenship', in Ong, S. and Collier, S.J. (eds) *Global Assemblages: Technology, Politics, and Ethics as Anthropological Problems,* Chichester: WileyBlackwell, pp. 439–63.

Rose, S (1997) *Lifelines: Life Beyond the Gene,* Oxford: Oxford University Press.

Routledge, P. (1996) 'The third space as critical engagement', *Antipode* 28 (4): 399–419.

——(2003) 'Convergence space: process geographies of grassroots globalization networks', *Transactions of the Institute of British Geographers* 28 (3): 333–49.

Royal Society (2003) *Keeping science open: the effects of intellectual property policy on the conduct of science,* London: Royal Society.

——(2004) *Nanoscience and nanotechnologies: opportunities and uncertainties* London: Royal Society.

SACGT (2001) *Development of a Classification Methodology for Genetic Tests,* Bethesda: SACGT.

Salter, B. and Jones, M. (2002) 'Regulating human genetics: the changing politics of biotechnology governance in the European Union', *Health, Risk and Society* 4 (3): 325–40.

Saukko, P., Richards, S., Shepherd, M. *et al.* (2006) 'Are genetic tests exceptional? Lessons from a qualitative study on thrombophilia', *Social Science & Medicine* 63 (7): 1947–59.

Savage, M. and Burrows, R. (2007) 'The coming crisis of empirical sociology', *Sociology* 41 (5): 885–99.

Saver, J.L. and Rabin, J. (1997) 'The neural substrates of religious experience', *Journal of Neuropsychiatry and Clinical Neurosciences* (1997) 9: 498–510.

Savulescu, J. (2001) 'Procreative beneficence: why we should select the best children', *Bioethics* 15: 413–26.

——(2004) 'Why we are morally obliged to genetically enhance our children' paper presented at First International Conference on Ethics, Science and Moral Philosophy of Assisted Human Reproduction, Royal Society, London, September 2004.

Schmitz, D., Henn, W. and Netzer, C. (2009) 'No risk, no objections? Ethical pitfalls of cell-free fetal DNA and RNA testing', *BMJ* 339: b2690.

Schneider, I. (2007) 'Indirect commodification of ova donation for assisted reproduction and for human cloning research – proposals for supranational regulation', in Steinmann, M., Skora, P. and Wiesing, U.(eds) *Altruism reconsidered: exploring new approaches to property in human tissue,* Aldershot: Ashgate.

Schneider, I and Schumann, C. (2002) 'Stem cells, therapeutic cloning, embryo research-Women as raw material suppliers for science and industry', in ReproKult, *Reproductive Medicine and Genetic Engineering: Women between Self-determination and Societal Standardisation,* Cologne: Federal Centre for Health Education.

Schramm, K. (2007) *Report on Research Stay at the University of Chicago,* Halle-Wittenberg: Martin-Luther-Universität.

Schroeder, D. (2007) 'Benefit sharing: it's time for a definition', *Journal of Medical Ethics* 33: 205–9.

Science (1998) 'Large-scale identification, mapping, and genotyping of single-nucleotide polymorphisms in the human genome', *Science* 280 (5366): 1077–82.

——(2008) 'Breakthrough of the year: reprogramming cells', *Science* 322 (5909): 1766–7.

Sen, J., Anita Anand, A., Escoba, A. and Waterman, P.(2004) *The World Social Forum: Challenging Empires,* New Delhi: Viveka Foundation.

Sexton, S. (1999) *If cloning is the answer, what was the question? Power and decision-making in the geneticization of health,* Sturminster Newton, Dorset: Corner House.

——(2002) 'Deceptive promises of cures for disease', *World-Watch* July 2002.

——(2005) 'Transforming "waste" into "resource": from women's eggs to economics for women', presented at ReproKult workshop 'Commodification and Commercialisation of Women's Bodies' at Femme Globale Conference, 10 September 2005.

Shiva, V. (1989) *Staying Alive: Women, Ecology and Survival in India,* London: Zed Press.

Silver, L.M.(1997) *Remaking Eden: How Genetic Engineering and Cloning Will Transform the American Family,* New York: Harper.

SIMR (2005) 'About SIMR' http://www.simr.org.uk/ (accessed 1 January 2005); SIMR (now PVMA) content no longer accessible.

Skene, L. (2001) 'Genetic secrets and the family: a response to Bell and Bennett', *Medical Law Review* 9 (2): 162–9.

Snow, D. and Benford, R. (1992) 'Master frames and cycles of Protest', in Morris, A.D. and Mueller, C. (eds) *Frontiers in Social Movement Theory,* New Haven, CT: Yale University Press.

Solanas, V. (1968) *The SCUM Manifesto (Society For Cutting Up Men),* Paris: Olympia Press.

SoR (2007) 'TUC: Society says "Genetic testing by employers and insurance companies must be regulated"', *Society of Radiographers News.*

Souza, A. (2003) 'People with Down's syndrome disrupt screening conference', *Inclusion Now* vol. 7.

Spallone, P. (1988) *Beyond Conception: The New Politics of Reproduction,* Basingstoke: Macmillan.

——(1992) *Generation Games: Genetic Engineering and the Future for Our Lives*, London: The Women's Press.

Stafford, M. and Marmot, M. (2003) 'Neighbourhood deprivation and health: does it affect us all equally?' *International Journal of Epidemiology* 32 (3) 357–66.

Stanley, L. (1991) 'Feminist auto/biography and feminist epistemology?' in Aaron, J. and Walby, S. (eds) *Out of the Margins; Women's Studies in the Nineties,* London: Falmer Press.

Star, S.L. and Griesemer, J.R. (1989). 'Institutional ecology, "translations" and boundary objects: amateurs and professionals in Berkeley's Museum of Vertebrate Zoology, 1907–39', *Social Studies of Science* 19 (3): 387–420.

Steinberg, M. (1998) 'Tilting the frame: Considerations on collective action framing from a discursive turn', *Theory and Society* 27(6): 845–72.

Sulston, J. and Ferry, G. (2002) *The Common Thread*, London: Bantam Press.

Sulston, J.E. and Horvitz, H.R. (1977) 'Post-embryonic cell lineages of the nematode, C. elegans', *Developmental Biology,* 56 (1):110–56.

Sun (2006) 'Docs to create mootant cells', 7 November 2006.

Szerszynski, B. (2005) 'Beating the unbound: political theatre in the laboratory without walls', in Giannachi, G. and Stewart, N., *Performing Nature: Explorations in Ecology and the Arts,* Frankfurt: Peter Lang.

TAC (2003) 'Settlement agreements secure access to affordable life-saving anti-retroviral medicines', *Treatment Action Campaign Newsletter* 10 December.

Tait, J. (2001) 'More Faust than Frankenstein: the European debate about the pre-cautionary principle and risk regulation for genetically modified crops', *Journal of Risk Research* 4 (2):175–89.

Tarrow, S. (1998) *Power in Movement: Social Movements, Collective Action, and Politics*, Cambridge: Cambridge University Press.

Telegraph, The Daily (2006) 'Volunteers never think it will happen to them', 16 March 2006, p. 10.

——(2008) 'UK biotech bosses call for Government rescue', 4 December.

The Age (2008) 'Controversial stem cell treatment draws Australians to Indian clinic', *The Age* 2 February.

Thomson, J., Itskovitz-Eldor, J., Shapiro, E. (1998). 'Embryonic stem cell lines derived from human blastocysts', *Science* 282 (5391): 1145–7.

Throsby, K. (2004) *When IVF Fails: Feminism, Infertility and the Negotiation of Normality*, Basingstoke: Palgrave.

Time (2008) 'Roche's Rush. How the Swiss firm is redefining the R& D crapshoot in its quest to land the next pharmaceutical breakthrough', 172 (15).

——(2009) 'Diabetes, heart disease, Parkinson's: how the coming revolution in stem cells could save your life', 9 February.

Times, The (2006) 'Junk medicine: therapeutic cloning – Science must milk the cow', 11 November.

——(2007) 'Discovery of "deaf gene" raises hopes of treatment', 18 June.

——(2008a) 'Animal-human embryo research is approved', 18 January.

——(2008b) 'David Cameron tells the fat and the poor: take responsibility', 8 July.

——(2008c) 'Postcode lottery of life and death', 28 August 2008.

——(2008d) 'European ruling could force "innocent" DNA samples to be removed from UK database', 4 December.

——(2008e) 'A stem bears fruit', 20 December.

——(2009) 'Parents to be offered test to detect inherited diseases in embryos', 1 July.

Torgersen, H., Jurgen Hampel, J. and von Bergmann-Winberg, M. *et al.* (2003) 'Promise, problems and proxies: twenty five years of debate and regulation in Europe', in Bauer, M.W. and Gaskell, G. (eds) *Biotechnology: The making of a global controversy,* Cambridge: Cambridge University Press.

Tormey, S. (2004) *Anticapitalism: A Beginner's Guide,* Oxford: Oneworld.

Tutton, R., Kerr, A. and Cunningham-Burley, S. (2005) 'Myriad stories: constructing expertise and citizenship in discussions of the new genetics', in Leach, M., Scoones, I. and Wynne, B.(eds) *Science and Citizens,* London: Zed Books.

UCL (ca. 2008) *Intercalated BSc Degree in Philosophy, Medicine, and Society,* London: University College.

UK Biobank (2007a) *Ethics and Governance Framework,* London: UK Biobank.

——(2007b) 'Invite letter', London: UK Biobank.

UKGTN (2008) *UK Genetic Testing Network: First Report,* London: UKGTN.

UKSCB (2004) *First Report from the UK Stem Cell Bank,* London: UK Stem Cell Bank.

UKSCF (2009) 'Stem cell research benefits and future hopes', (Brochure) London: UKSCF.

UN Wire (2002) 'NGOs begin meeting in Johannesburg', 19 August.

UNESCO (2002) *Human Genetic Data: Preliminary Study by the International Bioethics Committee on its Collection, Processing, Storage and Use,* Geneva: UNESCO.

——(2003) *International Declaration on Human Genetic Data,* Paris: UNESCO.

Uusitalo, S. (2008) 'Affective implications of GM food on social and individual integrity: an ethical approach', in Molfino, F. and Zucco, F. (eds) *Women in Biotechnology: Creating Interfaces,* New York: Springer.

Venter, J.C. (2007) *A Life Decoded. My Genome: My Life,* New York: Viking.

VHB (2008) 'Life-saving today. Life-changing tomorrow', (Brochure) London: Virgin Health Bank.

Wailoo, K. and Pemberton, S. (2006) *The Troubled Dream of Genetic Medicine: Ethnicity and Innovation in Tay-Sachs, Cystic Fibrosis, and Sickle Cell Disease,* Baltimore, MD: Johns Hopkins University Press.

Waldby, C. (2002) 'Stem cells, tissue cultures and the production of biovalue', *Journal for the Social Study of Health, Illness and Medicine* 6 (3): 305–23.

Wallace, H.M. (2006) 'A model of gene-gene and gene-environment interactions and its implications for targeting environmental interventions by genotype', *Theoretical Biology and Medical Modelling* (2006) 3: 35.

——(2008a) House of Lords Select Committee on Science and Technology, *Hansard* 9 July p. 8.

——(2008b) 'Most gene test sales are misleading', *Nature Biotechnology,* 26: 1221.

Warnock (1984) *Report of the Committee of Inquiry into Human Fertilisation and Embryology (the Warnock Report),* Cmd 9314, London: HMSO.

Watson, J.D. and Crick, F.H.C. (1953) 'A Structure for Deoxyribose Nucleic Acid', *Nature* 171 (4356): 737.

Wellcome (2004) *UK Biobank Ethics and Governance Framework,* London: Wellcome Foundation.

Welsh, I. (2000) *Mobilising Modernity: the Nuclear Moment,* London: Routledge.

Welsh, I., Plows, A. and Evans, R. (2007) 'Human rights and genomics: science, genomics and social movements at the 2004 London Social Forum', *New Genetics and Society* 26 (2): 123–35.

WHO (1946) *Constitution of the World Health Organization,* New York: World Health Organization.

——(2002) *Human Genetic Technologies: Implications for Preventive Health Care*, Geneva: World Health Organization.

——(2004) *Priorities for Research to Take Forward the Health Equity Policy Agenda*, Geneva: WHO.

——(2005) *Genetics, genomics and the patenting of DNA: Review of potential implications for health in developing countries*, Geneva: WHO.

Wikipedia (2009a) *DNA Sequencing* http://en.wikipedia.org/wiki/DNA_sequencing (accessed 8 June 2009).

——(2009b) *Diamond v. Chakrabarty, 447 U.S. 303 (1980), a United States Supreme Court case dealing with whether genetically modified micro-organisms can be patented* http://en.wikipedia.org/wiki/Diamond_v._Chakrabarty (accessed 9 June 2009).

Wilkinson, R.G (1996) *Unhealthy Societies: The Afflictions of Inequality*, London: Routledge.

Wilkinson, S. (2008) 'Sexism, sex selection and "family balancing"', *Medical Law Review* 16 (3): 369–89.

Wilsdon, J. and Willis, R. (eds) (2004) *See-through science; why public engagement needs to move 'upstream'*, London: Demos.

Wilsden, J. and Miller, P. (2006) *Better Humans*, London: Demos.

Wilson, E.O. (2000) *Sociobiology: The New Synthesis*, Cambridge, MA: Harvard University Press.

WIPO (2006) 'Bioethics and patent law: the case of myriad', *WIPO Magazine*.

WMA (2008) *Declaration of Helsinki*, Helsinki: World Medical Association.

Wolbring, G. (2006) 'The unenhanced underclass', in Miller, P. and Wilsdon, J. (eds). *Better Humans? The politics of human enhancement and life extension*, London: Demos.

Woyke, A. (2008) 'The world view of nanotechnology – philosophical reflections', in Jotterand, F. (ed.) *Emerging Conceptual, Ethical and Policy Issues in Bionanotechnology*, New York: Springer.

Wynne, B. (1996) 'May the sheep safely graze? A reflexive view of the expert–lay knowledge divide', in Lash, S., Szerszynski, B. and Wynne, B. (eds) *Risk, Environment & Modernity: Towards a New Ecology*, London: Sage.

——(2006) 'Public engagement as a means of restoring public trust in science – hitting the notes, but missing the music?' *Community Genetics* 2006 (9): 211–20.

Yeo, R. (2007) *'I don't have a problem, the problem is theirs': the priorities of Bolivian disabled people*, Leeds: Disability Press.

Index